Fabio Prosdocimi

New insights on serotonin and physical exercise

Fabio Prosdocimi

New insights on serotonin and physical exercise

Physical exercise activates the serotoninergic system

LAP LAMBERT Academic Publishing

Impressum/Imprint (nur für Deutschland/ only for Germany)
Bibliografische Information der Deutschen Nationalbibliothek: Die Deutsche Nationalbibliothek verzeichnet diese Publikation in der Deutschen Nationalbibliografie; detaillierte bibliografische Daten sind im Internet über http://dnb.d-nb.de abrufbar.
Alle in diesem Buch genannten Marken und Produktnamen unterliegen warenzeichen-, marken- oder patentrechtlichem Schutz bzw. sind Warenzeichen oder eingetragene Warenzeichen der jeweiligen Inhaber. Die Wiedergabe von Marken, Produktnamen, Gebrauchsnamen, Handelsnamen, Warenbezeichnungen u.s.w. in diesem Werk berechtigt auch ohne besondere Kennzeichnung nicht zu der Annahme, dass solche Namen im Sinne der Warenzeichen- und Markenschutzgesetzgebung als frei zu betrachten wären und daher von jedermann benutzt werden dürften.

Coverbild: www.ingimage.com

Verlag: LAP LAMBERT Academic Publishing GmbH & Co. KG
Dudweiler Landstr. 99, 66123 Saarbrücken, Deutschland
Telefon +49 681 3720-310, Telefax +49 681 3720-3109
Email: info@lap-publishing.com

Herstellung in Deutschland:
Schaltungsdienst Lange o.H.G., Berlin
Books on Demand GmbH, Norderstedt
Reha GmbH, Saarbrücken
Amazon Distribution GmbH, Leipzig
ISBN: 978-3-8443-1942-2

Imprint (only for USA, GB)
Bibliographic information published by the Deutsche Nationalbibliothek: The Deutsche Nationalbibliothek lists this publication in the Deutsche Nationalbibliografie; detailed bibliographic data are available in the Internet at http://dnb.d-nb.de.
Any brand names and product names mentioned in this book are subject to trademark, brand or patent protection and are trademarks or registered trademarks of their respective holders. The use of brand names, product names, common names, trade names, product descriptions etc. even without a particular marking in this works is in no way to be construed to mean that such names may be regarded as unrestricted in respect of trademark and brand protection legislation and could thus be used by anyone.

Cover image: www.ingimage.com

Publisher: LAP LAMBERT Academic Publishing GmbH & Co. KG
Dudweiler Landstr. 99, 66123 Saarbrücken, Germany
Phone +49 681 3720-310, Fax +49 681 3720-3109
Email: info@lap-publishing.com

Printed in the U.S.A.
Printed in the U.K. by (see last page)
ISBN: 978-3-8443-1942-2

TABLE OF CONTENTS

1. INTRODUCTION

1.1. Raphe nuclei

The raphe nuclei are the main neuronal clusters that synthesize serotonin (5-HT) in the central nervous system (CNS) (Dahlström, 1964; Björklund, 1971; Jacobs and Azmitia, 1992). Serotonin modulates somatic, neurovegetative, endocrine, and behavioral motor activity and its actions are dependent upon specific neuronal receptors that participate in a determined neuronal circuit (Parent, 1979; Aghajanian, 1985).

This nuclear complex consists of many neuronal cell clusters that can be divided into a number of smaller units based on their cytoarchitecture. They form a narrow cell column which extends along the median plane of the brainstem, from the caudal portion of the medulla oblongata to the interpeduncular nucleus of the mesencephalon. These nuclei are rostro-caudally named: rostral linear (RLi), caudal linear (CLi), dorsal (DR), median (MnR), paramedian (PMnR), pontine (PnR), magnus (RMg), pallidus (RPa) and obscurus (ROb) (Taber et al., 1977) (Figure 1). These clusters, besides forming local circuits in the reticular formation, have been divided into rostral and caudal nuclei that project, respectively, to structures of the prosencephalon and spinal cord.

The raphe nuclear complex possesses several similarities with the reticular formation itself (Taber et al., 1977). The assumption that the various raphe nuclei are distinct units is supported by anatomical and functional studies. However, due to their reduced dimensions, it is nearly impossible to study their individual connections and functions by means of electrical stimulation, neuronal lesion or neuronal tracer deposition.

Despite technical limitations, some studies on the functional importance of the rat raphe nuclei investigated the effects of discrete electrolytic lesions on behavior, which elicited deficits, such as insomnia, hyper-reactivity, aggression, and increases in pain and locomotor activity. However, large lesions encompassing several nuclei resulted in differential behavioral effects. Other functions have been attributed to the raphe nuclei, such as, motor (Holstege, 1982), endocrine (Smith, 1980), and visceral functions (Holstege, 1982), circadian rhythm modulation, learning and memory as well as somatic functions. Immunohistochemistry and immunofluorescent studies demonstrated that both noradrenergic (Morrison *et al.*, 1978) and 5-HTergic (Levitt *et al.*, 1984) fibers diffusely project to every region of the cerebral cortex exhibiting uniform fiber density, despite possessing variations in patterns of cortical arborization.

In an adult animal, the rostral linear (RLi) nucleus is the most rostral neuronal cluster, extending from 5.20 mm to 6.04 mm caudally to bregma. It is hypothesized that this nucleus acts as a chemosensor to substances circulating in the blood, possibly involved in the sleep/wake cycle (Brodal, 1984).

The caudal linear nucleus (CLi) is a neuronal cluster that initiates at 6.04 mm caudally from bregma, ventrally to the ventral tegmental decussation, extending up to 7.64 mm, ventral to the dorsal nucleus.

The dorsal (DR) is the largest raphe nucleus, containing approximately 40 percent of the 5-HTergic cells in the encephalon (Vertes and Kocsis, 1994). It is situated at the level of the rostral portion of the central gray matter (periaqueductal gray) and at nuclei below the fourth ventricle up to 9.30mm, caudally to bregma. It possesses the following subdivisions: caudal (DRC), dorsal (DRD),

4

ventrolateral (DRVL), ventral (DRV) and interfascicular subnucleus (DRI) (Baker, 1990). This dense 5-HTergic nucleus sends projections to other raphe nuclei (MnR, PnR, RMg and ROb), to structures of the mesencephalon and brainstem (mesencephalic reticular formation, lateral and medial parts of the parabrachial nucleus,oral part of the pontine reticular nucleus and *locus coeruleus*) as well as to the spinal cord, facial nucleus and hypoglossal nucleus (Vertes and Kocsis, 1994). The DR associated with REM sleep, regulation of neurovegetative functions via projections to the parabrachial complex and modulation of motosensory functions via projections to cranial nerves (Vertes and Kocsis, 1994). In addition, it is related to pain modulation (Wang and Nakai, 1994).

The median raphe nucleus (MnR), unlike other raphe nuclei, has well-defined limits in its rostro-medial portion in the pons, extending from the decussation of the superior cerebellar peduncle to the ventral tegmental nucleus. Anesthetized rats submitted to MnR electric stimulation exhibited increased pancreatic exocrine secretion and arterial blood pressure (Park, 1995). It sends projections to the suprachiasmatic nucleus (Tischler and Morin, 2003, Hay-Schimdt *et al.*, 2003) and to other raphe nuclei (ROb, RPa, RMg and DR), as well as to the hippocampal formation, laterodorsal tegmental nucleus, thalamic and hypothalamic regions (Vertes, 1999). It is possible to distinguish three cell groups in the MnR, dorsal, median and paramedian (Baker, 1990). Along with the DR nucleus, the MnR mediates cardiovascular control (Kaelher *et al.*, 2000).

The paramedian nucleus (PMnR) is located in the paramedian region, lateral to the MnR nucleus, extending from 7.64mm up to 8.30mm caudally to bregma.

The pontine nucleus (PnR) is a small neuronal cluster found in the rostral part of the pons, from the reticulotegmental nucleus to the beginning of the RMg. It receives projections from the raphe dorsal nucleus and has reciprocal connections with the *locus coeruleus* and cerebellum (Brodal, 1984).

The magnus nucleus (RMg) is present in the most rostral part of the medulla oblongata. In coronal sections, anatomically it has a triangular shape, positioned dorsally to the medial lemniscus, extending from the trapezoid body and following along the raphe obscurus nucleus. It is primarily related to analgesia modulation through inhibition of nociceptive neurons in the caudal part of the spinal trigeminal nucleus and in the posterior column of the spinal cord (Bowker, 1986; Carpenter, 1991). In addition, the RMg also participates in frenic nerve activity (Smith, 1980). It has projections to vestibular nuclei (Halberstadt and Balaban, 2003) and is related to pain modulation during sleep (Foo and Mason, 2003).

The raphe pallidus nucleus (RPa) extends caudally from bregma point at 9.56mm to the pyramidal decussation. It represents a dense neuronal cluster found between the pyramids, close to the ventral surface of the medulla oblongata. Along with the obscurus nucleus, this nucleus constitutes the main 5-HTergic afferent to the motor trigeminal nucleus, acting as facilitatory relay (Ribeiro do Valle, 1997). It also projects to facial and hypoglossal nuclei (Holstege and Kyupers, 1987), as well as to vestibular nuclei, although in smaller densities when compared with the DR nucleus (Halberstadt and Balaban, 2003).

The obscurus nucleus (Rob) has neurons situated in two paramedian clusters, extending caudally from bregma at 11.16mm to the pyramidal decussation end. It is ventrally limited by the inferior olive and dorsally by the fourth ventricle. It also has projections to the vestibular nuclei (Halberstadt and Balaban, 2003) and is mainly related to locomotor activity (Jacobs and Fornal, 1993).

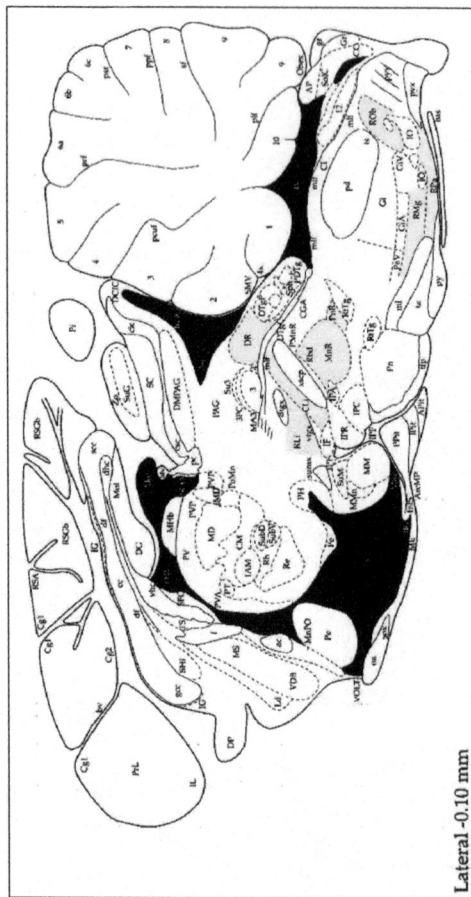

Lateral -0.10 mm

Figure 1. Sagittal section of rat brain (0.10mm lateral) exhibiting raphe nuclei, highlighted in yellow (modified from Paxinos and Watson, 1998).

1.2. Reticular formation

The reticular formation *"is a continuous small group of isodendritic cells which crosses the brainstem, from the spinal intermediate reticular gray layers to the subthalamus, parts of the hypothalamus, and of the dorsal thalamus"* (Willians *et al.*, 1989). This area consists of:

1- Groups of poorly defined neurons and fibers with diffuse connections deeply situated in the brainstem;

2- Poorly defined neuronal pathways, revealed by physiological evidence;

3- Ascending and descending connections which are partially contralateral and ipsilateral, showing bilateral response to unilateral stimuli;

4- Somatic and visceral connections.

The brainstem reticular formation is structurally characterized by areas comprised of diffuse clusters of neurons exhibiting different types and sizes, separated by a profusion of fibers traveling in all directions. Certain circular-shaped adjacent nuclei, such as the red nucleus and cranial nerve nuclei are not included. Thus, the most frequently used criterion to consider a cellular area as part of the reticular formation is its structure. Therefore, the term "reticular formation" will be used to name areas of the brainstem (mesencephalon, pons and medulla oblongata) that have a reticular structure, except nuclei (paramedian reticular nucleus, reticulotegmental nucleus of the pons and lateral reticular nucleus) that project to the cerebellum.

The reticular formation area considered here encompasses central areas of the brainstem. Therefore, peripherally, each half of the reticular formation is limited by long bundles of ascending and descending fibers crossing the brainstem (medial longitudinal fascicle, medial lemniscus, spinothalamic tract), and by determined nuclei that may invade part of its territory (Brodal, 1984).

There are cytoarchitectural differences in the reticular formation of different species, and the boundaries across groups are not always evident. Besides, the limits between the reticular formation and certain nuclei, for example, the vestibular and trigeminal sensory nuclei, are not well defined. Therefore, there are vast architectural differences across relatively small areas of the reticular formation. Other differences between these areas of the reticular formation, such as connections and function, could be considered. An evident characteristic is that large cells of the reticular formation are restricted to its medial part, where they blend with small and medium cells, whereas in the lateral third there are only small cells.

Cytoarchitectural studies on the reticular formation by the Golgi method provided additional information about its cellular, dendritic, and axonal patterns. All axons seem to project, at least to a certain extent, rostrally and/or caudally. Reticular cell dendrites are usually radial and long (Ramón-Moliner and Nauta, 1966), and it is typical that dendrites be displayed in a perpendicular plane along the brainstem axis (Brodal, 1984).

There are some smaller cell groups, which, despite their reticular structure, have been specifically named and are not included in the reticular formation. However, since these nuclei are similar to other parts of the reticular formation with similar connections, it is very probable that they are functionally correlated to it. This is the case of the raphe nuclei, associated with motricity (Brodal, 1984) and analyzed in this study.

1.3. Exercise and Physical Conditioning

Today, there is increased awareness of the benefits of exercise and physical activity, primarily with respect to health improvement. There is evidence to show that physical activity reduces the risk of chronic diseases and premature death, besides offering better quality of life (Dishman, 2003). After the publication of *Physical Activity and Health: A Report of the Surgeon General* (US Department of Health and Human Services, 1990), years of research on exercise and physical activity finally promoted the concept of the physiology of exercise as a multidisciplinary science (Raven, 1989). Exercise promotes beneficial effects on brain function, improving neuronal plasticity and increasing both memory performance and learning (Tong, 2001). Decreased depression indices as well as improved mental health were evidenced in subjects who engage in physical exercise when compared to sedentary subjects (Dishman, 2003).

Studies carried out with the implementation of physical activity programs in the workplace demonstrated that for each American dollar spent; approximately $3.40 was saved, resulting in cost savings from reduced medical expenses and hospitalizations (Gettman, 1996).

Prolonged exercises at low-to-moderate intensity are characterized by 60% to 80% of the maximum heart rate, thus using aerobic metabolism as its energy source (Pollock and Schadwick, 1994).In particular, aerobic exercise helps reduce body fat and preserves muscle mass (Pollock, 1993).

In fact, sedentarism or physical inactivity is a factor linked to numerous pathologies, such as coronaropathy and colon cancer (Prochaska and Diclemente, 1983; Pate *et al.*, 1995), and is associated with the development of hypertension, one of the major risk factors for stroke (Blair *et al.*, 1984, Wells, 1996). However, physical activity is associated with a reduced incidence of colon cancer (Lee, 1995), with a significant mortality reduction in individuals who are engaged in moderate physical activity (Wells, 1996). Regular physical activity also reduces the risk for type 2 diabetes by 25% because it consumes from 1.500 to 2000 Kcal (Helmrich et a.l, 1991) and is associated with mental health improvement (Dishman, 1998).

Moderate regular exercises may elevate the immune response against infectious agents in athletes and individuals who exercise (Mackinnon, 2000). This relation between the effects of physical exercise and its benefits to the immune system has been described and investigated by several authors who support the hypothesis that such results are a consequence of immunomodulation (Pedersen, 1997).

Exercise also stimulates the production of pre-inflammatory cytokines and lymphocytes, increasing the chance of recovery following myocardial infarction in rats (Bassit et al., 2000). Exercise prevents many of the behavioral and physiological consequences derived from stress. Physical exercise has been proposed to improve the general health of individuals with varied health problems, where beneficial effects can be obtained through complex interactions between psychological and physiological effects, such as stress relief, improvement of cardiovascular function, and metabolic stabilization. Thus, physical exercise facilitates an increase in oxidative capacity, body fat reduction, and hormonal modulation (Brines *et al.*, 1996). It has also been described that physical exercise can potentiate vaccine efficiency; for example, against tuberculosis (BCG, Bacillus Calmette-Guerin), by increasing the IgG antibody (Martins, 2009).

With respect to the adequate dose of physical activity for each individual, it is worth highlighting that the optimal level of exercise for each individual is different, therefore some factors must be taken into consideration. According to the American College of Sports Medicine – (ACSM, 1978), an adequate training model consists of:

a- Training frequency of 3 to 5 days per week;

b- Training duration of 15 to 60 minutes;

c- Rhythmic and aerobic use of large muscle groups.

According to the ACSM, "Children and adults alike should set a goal of accumulating at least 30 minutes of moderate-intensity physical activity on most, and preferably all days of the week" (NIH Consensus Development Panel on Physical activity and Cardiovascular Health, 1995; Pate et al., 1995; U.S. Department of Health and Human Services,1996; American Heart Association, 1996).

One should still consider that the frequency and duration of physical exercise is fundamental to obtain these beneficial results. Duration refers to the time extension of the performance period of each training session (amount of minutes or hours). Frequency refers to the number of times each training session is performed (Jackson et al., 1968; Pollock et al., 1969; Knuttgen et al., 1973; Fox et al., 1975; Gettman, 1976). A training sequence recommended in an aerobic program is three to five times a week, and the more prolonged and more frequent the training session is, the better the results will be (Fox et al., 1973). However, taking into consideration physiological and performance aspects, there is no scientific evidence that increased daily training sessions increase aptitude benefits (Watt et al., 1973; Mostardi et al., 1975; Costill et al., 1991). The adequate training model mentioned above has been adopted because it considers parameters of: a) energy supply and depletion; b) muscle potential; c) biomechanics; d) and physiology. These parameters had not been previously addressed by pioneer physiologists, such as Hill, Bock and Drill (Noakes, 2000).

It is worth mentioning that our body works like an integrated system, and during physical training sessions an involvement of the neuromuscular system, skeletal muscle system, and cardiovascular system occurs, determining power and endurance during prolonged periods of time. Some factors influence and determine performance, such as movement endurance, oxygen consumption value (VO_2), maximum oxygen consumption value (VO_2 max), lactate threshold and energy conservation (Pate, 1992; Coyle, 1995). Given that these factors only indicate adequate performance, they will not be addressed in this book. There are several types of endurance training regimens; however we will only investigate prolonged moderate-intensity training (Pate and Branch, 1992).

Prolonged moderate-intensity training consists of 30 minutes to two hours of long-distance running, sometimes designated as long slow distance (LSD) (Daniels *et al.*, 1978). The training model adopted in the present study was swimming, following the moderate-intensity swimming protocol.

In the overall population, the risk of sudden death during exercise is small; approximately one in every 100.000 people. However, its occurrence is generally widely reported in the media, jeopardizing the message of the benefits of physical conditioning programs (American Heart Association, 1992; Kohl, 1992). This statistic is higher than that found during inactive periods, clearly indicating a transitory increase in the risk of sudden death. However, it is important to mention that the risk of sudden death during exercise is higher in sedentary individuals than in habitually active individuals (Mittleman *et al.*, 1993). Thus, the benefits touted by a physical activity program are favorable when aimed at lowering the global risk of sudden death. In the Unites States, 10 to 12 percent of the population exercises regularly; 15 percent of the population exercises to improve health, but this does not translate to a great impact due to a deficiency in the physical activity program; 30 percent exercise irregularly and 40 percent are completely sedentary. In general, approximately 60 percent of the population is at a level where physical activity is not being performed at the recommended frequency, duration, or intensity to obtain the ideal quality of life and health. This percentage is even higher for individuals who smoke at least one pack of cigarettes a day, or those who possess systolic arterial pressure higher or equal to 150 mmHg or who possess cholesterol levels higher than 265 mg/dl. Interestingly, the drop out rate for regular physical activity programs is quite similar to drop out rates for psychotherapy, weight loss, and drug and tobacco abuse programs (Dishman, 2003).

1.4. Muscle control and fatigue

Muscle contraction results from the movement of myosin over actin microfilaments, determining muscle shortening. This shortening is dependent upon certain factors, such as: a) ATP decomposition and energy release; b) Ca^{2+} binding to troponin, activating actin microfilaments; c) actomyosin formation (myosin and actin complex).

The motor neuron and all the muscle fibers to which it connects constitute a functional unit known as motor unit, which works to determine contraction. Thus, it is possible to modulate the degree of contraction strength of a muscle group by:

a) alternating the contraction frequency of single motor units, a factor known as wave summation;

b) recruiting or adding multiple motor units, that is, varying the number of contracted motor units at a certain moment, a factor known as motor unit summation.

There are different muscle fibers, basically Type I (slow twitch) or Type II (fast twitch). A motor unit does not have both fiber types together. Type II fibers can be further categorized into Type IIA, Type IIB and Type IIC fibers. Type I fibers have higher aerobic capacity, Type IIA are both glycolytic and oxidative, Type IIB have an anaerobic glycolytic metabolism and Type IIC present no classification or differentiation (Goldspink, 1985). There is a consensus that the volume increase of a muscle is due to hypertrophy and not to hyperplasia (Gollnick *et al.*, 1981). When comparing endurance athletes (distance runners) to athletes who lift weight, the latter present lower percentage of Type I fibers and higher percentage of Type IIA and IIB fibers, as well as larger number of mitochondria and lower intracellular lipid content within muscle fibers (Staron *et al.*, 1984, Miller *et al.*, 1995).

It is worth clarifying that the fiber type predominant during pregnancy is the undifferentiated Type IIC.

The differentiation of Type IIC fibers from Type I, IIA and IIB fibers occurs as the maturation of the muscle and nervous systems takes place, when axial and appendicular muscles begin to work. After birth, an increase in Type I fibers, important for locomotion and endurance, is observed. Later, Type I and II fibers are relatively equivalent, modifying fiber diameter during the second decade of life (Vogler and Bove, 1985). It has been demonstrated by means of cross-innervation of different fiber types (I and II), that the motor nerve is responsible for defining functional muscle capacity

(Munsat *et al.*, 1976; Gordon and Pattullo, 1993; Talmadge *et al.*, 1993).

When muscle fibers are repeatedly activated, energy-consuming processes occur (ATP) and the muscle gets tired, producing less force. Once fatigued, muscle fibers take longer to relax, as relaxation is an active process which requires energy (ATP). Given that, longer relaxation periods permit that force produced by repeated nerve impulses be added even at low frequencies (longer intervals between action potentials), when compared with the muscle at rest (Kandel *et al.*, 2003).

Local muscular contractile fatigue, signal the encephalon to inhibit the motor system via inhibitory efferents mediating muscle performance reduction; therefore, when the muscle fatigues, afferent impulses are conveyed to the CNS.

In motor areas of the CNS, fatigue influences the muscle response to exercise and can be defined as "a reduction in the muscle force derived from the decline in the motor neuron activity" (Gandevia *et al.*, 1995) or as loss of force-generating capacity (Nybo, 2003). 5-HT receptors are fatigue-determining factors in motor areas of the CNS (Dwyer and Browning, 2000). There is extensive evidence that 5-HT plays a fundamental role in CNS-mediated fatigue during prolonged physical exercise. The 5-HT functions related to the sleep-wake cycle, lethargy and motricity suggest that 5-HT is a probable neuromediator of the central fatigue mechanism (Newsholme *et al.*, 1987). Physical exercise may influence important factors that control 5-HT synthesis and reuptake in the CNS in such a way that increased brain 5-HT levels during prolonged exercise may lead to central fatigue, thus, impairing physical activity performance (Newsholme and Blomstrand, 1996). The increase in brain 5-HT levels occurs as a response to the increase in tryptophan (Trp) concentration, the amino acid precursor to 5-HT. Most of the Trp present in the plasma is bound to albumin; however free tryptophan (f-Trp) is transported past the blood-brain barrier. This transport occurs via specific receptors which share Trp with other amino acids, more specifically the branched-chain amino acids (BCAAs) leucine, isoleucine and valine. Consequently, brain 5-HT synthesis increases with higher concentrations of f-Trp in blood plasma in relation to the total plasma concentration of BCAA (i.e. when f-Trp/BCAA rises). This increase was observed during prolonged exercise due to two factors: first BCAAs are initially taken up from the blood and oxidized during skeletal muscle contraction; and second, fatty acid (FA) concentration increases, mediating an increase in plasma f-Trp, once it releases Trp from albumin binding sites (Davis *et al.*, 2000).

If an individual pauses between exercises, muscle disorders tend to decrease. For example, if a person performs a dispersive activity in between exercise, for instance book reading, signs from different regions will reach facilitatory brain areas. Consequently, facilitating impulses activate the locomotor system, determining fast fatigue recovery (Asmussen and Mazin, 1978).

A neural network able to generate a rhythmic pattern of neural activity is called a central pattern generator (CPG), which occurs due to the interaction of cellular properties and synaptic connections (Kiehn *et al.*, 1997; Calabrese *et al.*, 1998) related to various locomotor patterns, including swimming. The CPG basically depends on three factors:

a- Individual neuronal characteristics;

b- Synaptic properties between neurons;

c- Inhibition and excitation of interconnected neurons.

This neural network is sensitive to 5-HTergic pharmacological stimulation, as demonstrated in the rat spinal cord, region responsible for the basic circuit to generate CPG (Ribotta *et al.*, 2000). The spinal cord contains neuronal circuits which mediate automatic and reflex movements, such as locomotion. The brainstem possesses similar circuits for face and mouth reflex movements. The motor cortex (like the premotor cortex) performs the highest level of motor control. The motor cortex projects directly to the spinal cord through the corticospinal tract and modulates motor tracts originated in the brainstem.

The cerebellum and basal nuclei also participate in the regulation, planning and execution of movement through reward circuits which regulate motor and premotor cortices and brainstem areas, receiving afferents from cortical areas and projecting to motor cortical areas through the thalamus (Grillner, 1981; Belanger *et al.*, 1988).

When the motor cortex is stimulated, specific motor and sympathetic neurovegetative effects related to somatic and general adaptation to exercise performance are triggered (Paulus and Geyer, 1993). The caudal hypothalamus sends projections to motor areas and to the RPa, while medial portions of the hypothalamus and of the preoptic region project to the RMg (Holstege, 1995).

Motor neuron cell bodies that innervate individual muscles are clustered in motor nuclei, arranged in longitudinal columns. These columns extend from one to four spinal segments, following a progressive spatial order rule in the interior of the spinal cord, where motor nuclei innervating the most proximal muscles situate more medially than those innervating the most distal muscles (Kandel *et al.*, 2003).

A characteristic aspect of voluntary movements is its performance improvement with practice, possibly associated with cortical reorganization. Image mapping by cortical magnetic resonance imaging (MRI) demonstrated that the cortical area activated during the performance of a training sequence was larger than that activated during a non-trained sequence (Le Bihan and Karni, 1995).

Intense muscle exercise is an efficient stimulus to activate Fos (*Finkel-Birkis-Jinkins murine osteosarcoma*) protein expression, a metabolic neuronal marker in the CNS.

1.5. Fos

The Fos protein is a product of the homologous proto-oncogenec *fos,* one of the immediate early expression genes of the oncogene *v-fos*, observed in the virus that causes a type of osteosarcoma (Curran and Teich, 1982). It is rapidly induced in neurons after efficient external stimuli (Morgan and Curran, 1989), reaching its highest nuclear concentration within approximately 60-90 minutes (Morgan and Curran, 1991; Krukoff, 1993; Rowland, 1996; Dinardo, 1997) and persisting for 2 to 5 hours (Draisci and Iadarola, 1989). Therefore, FOS protein is a nuclear phosphoprotein that marks neuronal activity during specific stimulation, and can be employed as an efficient method of mapping neuronal circuits in the CNS during physiological activity.

There is a sequence of events that culminate with Fos production. Initially, efficient extracellular stimulation opens calcium channels enabling these ions to enter the cell (Figure 2), activating CaM (Ca^{2+}/calmodulin) kinase II, which is responsible for the phosphorilation of the transcription factor CREB (cAMP response element binding protein, a binding protein responsive to cAMP). CREB has a phosphorylation-activation site and a motif for

DNA binding. Therefore, when activated via cAMP, CREB binds to the CREB response element (CRE), initiating the transcription of c-fos and Jun B immediate early genes, producing Fos and Jun proteins. Both have a leucine zipper-like motif, which is composed of a region with approximately 30 amino acids and characterized by repeats of leucine for every seven amino acids. The leucine motifs of the two proteins form dimers with α-parallel helices. Thus, Jun and Fos dimerize to form a heterodimer, the AP-1 complex. This dimerazation increases the affinity for activation and repression domains (Figure 2). Thus, several DNA portions containing the specific site for this factor are activated, modulating neurotransmitter synthesis.

Fos protein can be visualized by the immunohistochemistry method, through labeled neuron nuclei; thus, immunohistochemistry is a valuable technique for anatomical and physiological combined studies to identify Fos expression in the CNS, induced by peripheral stimuli.

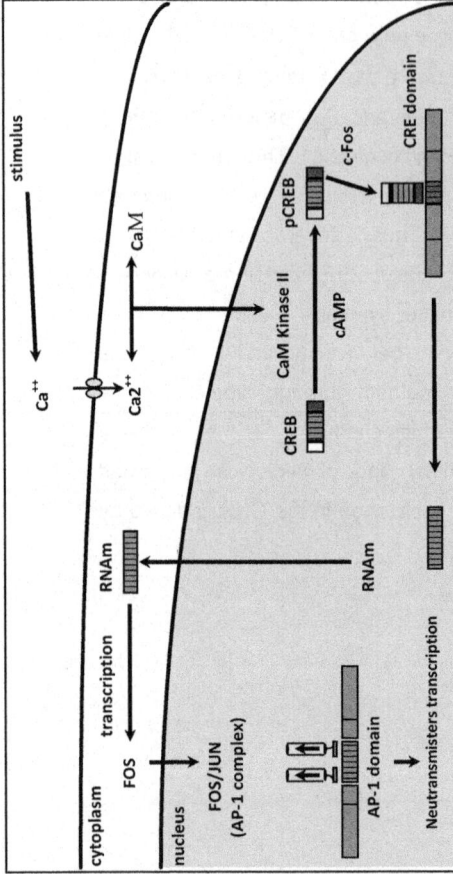

Figure 2. Stimulated receptor opens Ca^{2+} channels. Once in the cytoplasm, it activates Ca^{2+}/calmodulin (CaM) kinase II enzyme, which then phosphorilates CREB transcription factor, which in turn induces proto-oncogene *c-fos* expression when binding to CRE DNA binding site. Fos protein dimerizes with another protein (Jun) to form the AP-1 complex heterodimer, which will modulate transcription of genes that possess the AP-1 binding site (modified from Honrado *et al.*, 1996; Takase *et al.*, 2000).

2. PROPOSITION

Verify the involvement of raphe nuclei and their potential anatomical and functional alterations resulting from homeostatic responses of animals submitted to physical exercises compared to results from sedentary animals. For this, immunohistochemistry was used to quantify neurons expressing Fos in different raphe nuclei and their distribution along the rostrocaudal axis of each animal within different experimental groups.

3. MATERIAL AND METHODS

3.1. Animals

Fifteen albino (*Ratus norwegicus*, Wistar), three-month-old male rats, weighing from 290- 320g were maintained under controlled temperature (23° C), 12/12h light/dark cycle (lights on at 07:00h) with food and water available *ad libtum*. The animals were divided into two groups: trained (group T, n=9), which were submitted to the moderate-intensity swimming protocol for eight weeks, and sedentary (group S, n=6), which received no physical training. All procedures followed the guidelines from the *International Guiding Principles for Biomedical Research Involving Animals* (Society for Neuroscience, 1991), Brazilian College of Animal Experimentation (Cobea, 1991) and were approved by the Local Ethical Committee for Animal Research (Biomedical Sciences Institute, São Paulo University, SP, Brazil).

3.2. Experimental conditions – Moderate-intensity swimming protocol

Group T animals were submitted to a moderate-intensity swimming protocol developed by Lancha Júnior *et al.*

(1997) for eight weeks (Table 1), from 12:00 to 13:00h, following five days of training and two days of rest.

A system of ten isolated plastic tanks was used for the training sessions (Figure 3). To avoid competition and minimize stress, the animals could not see each other (Figure 4).

Moderate-intensity swimming training protocol				
	Monday	Tuesday	Wednasday	Thursday	Friday
Week 1	T: 15' SC: 0%	T: 20' SC: 0%	T: 30' SC: 0%	T: 40' SC: 1%	T: 40' SC: 2%
Week 2	T: 50' SC: 2%	T: 50' SC: 3%	T: 60' SC: 3%	T: 50' SC: 4%	T: 60' SC: 4%
Week 3	T: 40' SC: 5%	T: 50' SC: 5%	T: 60' SC: 5%	T: 60' SC: 5%	T: 60' SC: 5
Week 4	T: 60' SC: 5%	T: 60' SC: 5%	T: 60' SC: 5%	T: 60' SC: 5%	T: 60' SC: 5%
Week 5	T: 60' SC: 5%	T: 60' SC: 5%	T: 60' SC: 5%	T: 60' SC: 5%	T: 60' SC: 5%
Week 6	T: 60' SC: 5%	T: 60' SC: 5%	T: 60' SC: 5%	T: 60' SC: 5%	T: 60' SC: 5%
Week 7	T: 60' SC: 5%	T: 60' SC: 5%	T: 60' SC: 5%	T: 60' SC: 5%	T: 60' SC: 5%
Week 8	T: 60' SC: 5%	T: 60' SC: 5%	T: 60' SC: 5%	T: 60' SC: 5%	T: 60' SC: 5%

Table 01. Moderate-intensity swimming training protocol (Lancha Júnior et al., 1997).

Note: T1 – T9, animals submitted to training; S1 – S6, sedentary animals.

T, training time in minutes.

AW, additional weight added to animal's tail.

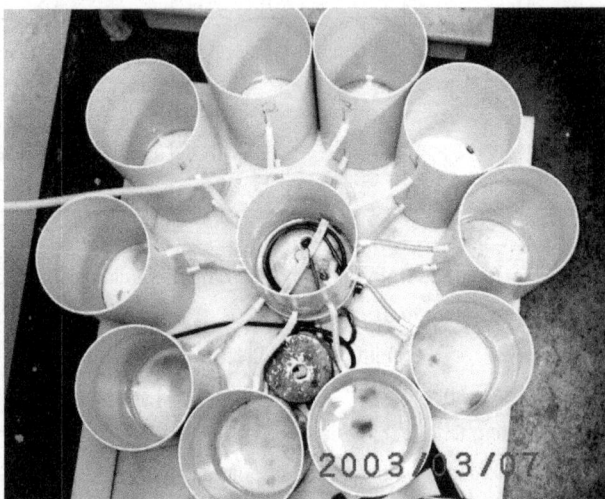

Figure 3. System of ten isolated plastic tanks used for training sessions.

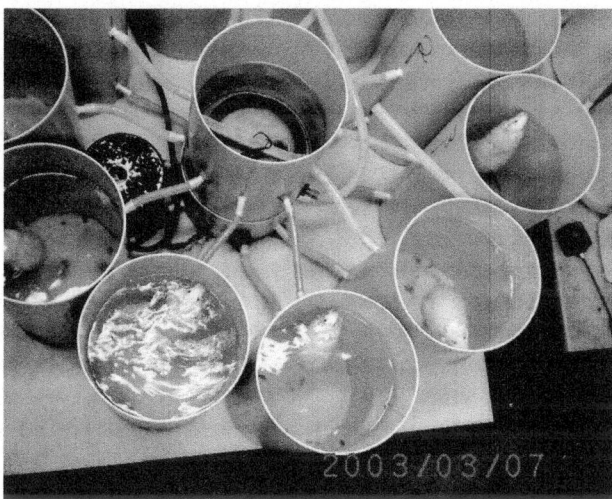

Figure 4. Animals during training.

The water volume in each tank was sufficient to prevent the animal's tail from touching the tank bottom. This was an important technical consideration in the training protocol, since it prevented the animals from decreasing their swimming effort, which could invalidate the moderate-intensity swimming protocol.

The tank water was changed after each training session and the temperature was measured before and after each session (temperature between 30-32ºC). After training, animals were transferred to a cage, dried to remove excess water and placed in the animal room. During training, additional weights were added to the animals (Figure 5). The addition of weight is necessary since animals usually adapt to physical exercises during the experiment and are likely to progressively use less effort.

Group S animals did not receive any training and were sacrificed following one single moderate-intensity swimming session, using the same session duration as group T animals. These animals were previously submitted to adaptation of the experimental environment. The adaptation consisted of placing the animal in the training tank for 30 minutes for one week, with enough water to allow environmental adaptation, aiming to minimize stress-induced activation at sacrifice. The Group S swimming session was carried out at the same time as group T and no weights were added, as there was not enough time for exercise adaption.

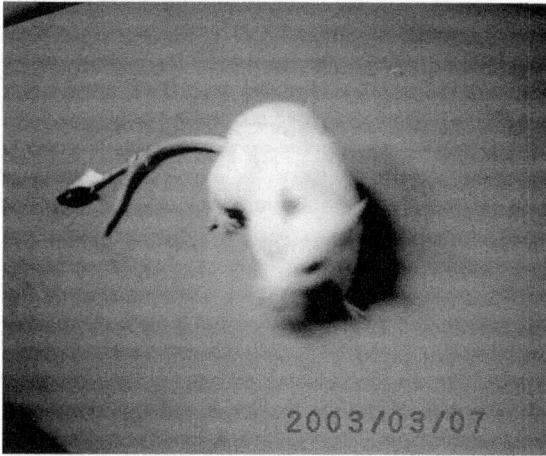

Figure 5. Weight added to animal's tail.

3.3. Specimen Preparation

Animals were sacrificed by perfusion as previously described 90 min after completion of the training regimen, to obtain maximum Fos protein expression (Laudanna et al., 1998). Firstly, animals were deeply anesthetized with intraperitoneal injection of 3% pentobarbital and the thoracic cavity was exposed. An intracardiacinjection of heparin was administered to avoid blood clotting. The aorta was cannulated using a peristaltic pump system. The descending aorta was clamped, so that during perfusion the fixative solution would not reach the abdomen and lower extremities, guaranteeing better fixation of the animal brain and using less fixative. The animals were initially perfused with 150 ml of 0.9% NaCl solution at room temperature for 2 min to remove blood from the vascular system. Animals were then perfused with 500 ml of 4% paraformaldehyde in 0.1 M sodium tetraborate buffer, pH 9.5, at 4°C for 5 minutes at rapid flow, followed by 15 minutes at slow flow. The rapid initial fixative solution flow is important to allow quick tissue preservation, diminishing protein degradation, and the slow flow allows more formaldehyde molecules to reach the tissues. The tetraborate sodium buffer acts as a protein protector, minimizing protein degradation during the tissue fixation process. When muscle contraction of the upper extremities and head was observed due to penetration of the fixative solution in the tissues, the animal's head was immediately covered with ice to minimize protein degradation.

The brains were then carefully dissected out and removed, post-fixed in the same fixative solution supplemented with 20% sucrose for 4 hours at 4°C. The brains were further cryoprotected in potassium phosphate buffered saline (KPBS) supplemented with 20% sucrose overnight at 4°C and, cryosectioned coronally at a thickness of 40 μm. The sections were collected in 1-in-5 series and stored in antifreeze solution (0.05 M sodium phosphate buffer supplemented with 30% ethylene-glycol and 20% glycerol) in a -20°C freezer.

3.4. Immunohistochemistry

One series of brain sections was submitted to Fos protein immunodetection by the immunoperoxidase method using ABC (Avidin-Biotin Complex) and diaminobenzidine chromogen (DAB). The sections were mounted on gelatin-coated slides and intensified with osmium tetroxide. An adjacent series of brain sections was submitted to the Nissl method using thionin, for cytoarchitectural references.

The detailed procedures for Fos immunoperoxidase detection in the brain sections were as follows:

1) Three rinses in 0.02 M KPBS, pH 7.4 for 10 min;

2) Incubation in 30% H_2O_2 solution to reduce background labeling by neutralizing endogenous peroxidases;

3) Three rinses in KPBS for 10 min;

4) Incubation in 1% sodium borohydride solution in KPBS to remove groups of free aldehydes;

5) Several rinses in KPBS, until bubbles disappear from brain sections;

6) Incubation in rabbit polyclonal anti-Fos primary antibody against the N-terminal synthetic peptide fragment (Oncogene Science Inc., USA) at 1:10000 for 48 h at 4°C (Hoffman, 2002). The antibody was diluted in a KPBS, Triton X-100 (0.3%) and normal goat serum (1:50) solution. Triton X-100 facilitates antibody penetration in the tissue and normal goat serum inactivates non-specific sites for secondary antibody binding;

7) Three rinses in KPBS for 10 min;

8) Incubation in biotinylated secondary antibody diluted in KPBS supplemented with Triton X-100 (0.3%) and normal goat serum (1:50), for 90 min at room temperature.

9) Three rinses in 0.1 M sodium acetate buffer solution, pH 6.0, for 10 min;

10) Incubation in avidin-biotin complex (ABC) diluted in KPBS for 90 min. Avidin possesses four biotin binding sites, one of them binds to the secondary antibody biotin and the others are filled by free biotin charged with peroxidase molecules;

11) Three rinses in KPBS for 10 min;

12) Incubation with DAB chromogen (3-3'-diaminobenzidine tetrahydrochloride) in 0.1 M sodium acetate buffer supplemented with 5% nickel and ammonium sulphate, glucose oxidase, β-D (+) glucose and 0.04% ammonium chloride. Note that the peroxidase reaction is more efficient when it occurs at pH 6.0. Peroxide (H_2O_2) originates from the reaction between glucose oxidase and β-D (+) glucose, with ammonium chloride as a catalyst.

13) Peroxidase inactivation through incubation in 0.1M sodium acetate buffer;

14) Three rinses in KPBS for 10 min;

15) Mounting of brain sections on gelatin-coated slides and overnight air drying at room temperature.

After the immunohistochemistry reaction, the brain slides were submitted to osmication procedure in order to intensify immunolabeling. For this, slides were submitted to dehydration and hydration sequences using ethanol and xylene; immersed in 0.005% osmium tetroxide and in 0.05% thiocarbohydrazide solutions, for 15 min each. The slides were then rinsed in tap water for 15 minutes and reimmersed in 0.005% osmium tetroxide solution for 30 min, dehydrated in increasing concentrations of ethanol and xylene. Finally, the slides were coverslipped using DPX as a non-aqueous mounting medium.

3.5. Analysis of results

The brain slides were analyzed under a light microscope (Axioplan, Leica, Germany) coupled to a digital camera and a computer system with image analysis software (Image-Pro Plus v.6, Media Cybernetics Inc, MD, USA) to quantify labeled neurons (Fos-immunoreactive, Fos-IR) in the raphe nuclei. A Fos-IR neuron counting pattern was established for each animal using the rat brain stereotaxic atlas (Paxinos and Watson, 1998) and the adjacent series of Nissl-stained brain slides. Only neurons with evident nuclear labeling were considered for counting (Figure 06). The Fos-IR neuronal number was expressed as means with standard deviation (SD) and/or standard error (SE) for each brain region.

3.6. Statistical analysis

Data were computed and submitted to analysis of variance (ANOVA) and Tukey´s *post-hoc* test, considering $P<0.05$ as significant.

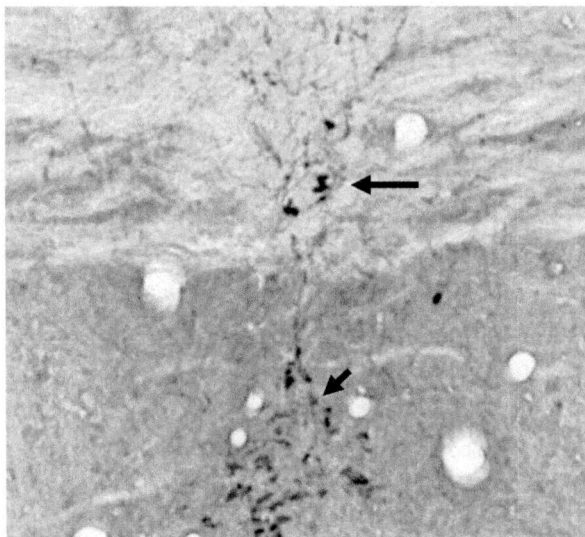

Figure 6. Bright-field photomicrograph of caudal linear nucleus of the raphe (CLi), approximately 5.96mm caudally from bregma. Note the neurons exhibiting nuclei with discrete labeling (small arrow) and dense labeling (large arrow). (100x original magnification).

4. RESULTS

This study observed the neuronal activation of different raphe nuclei by Fos immunodetection in trained and sedentary animals. The main results are presented below.

4.1. Body weight

The mean weight of animals submitted to the moderate-intensity swimming protocol was lower than that observed in sedentary animals, culminating in fat tissue reduction (Table 2).

Animal #	Week 1	Week 2	Week 3	Week 4	Week 5	Week 6
T1	180	195	215	230	250	280
T2	185	200	215	235	245	280
T3	175	190	220	235	250	275
T4	190	205	220	240	255	280
T5	190	205	225	240	250	275
T6	195	210	220	245	255	270
T7	180	200	220	235	250	280
T8	195	205	225	235	255	280
T9	200	215	225	235	245	270
S1	180	200	225	250	275	305
S2	190	210	230	245	275	305
S3	190	215	235	250	280	310
S4	190	210	235	245	290	320
S5	185	210	240	255	285	320
S6	185	215	235	255	285	325

Table 2. Body weight monitoring. T1 to T9, trained animals; S1 to S6, sedentary animals.

4.2. Microscopic analysis

The dorsal raphe nucleus (DR) had 56.67 ± 1.39 (mean ± SD) Fos-IR neuronsin group T(increase of 29.76%) compared to group S (47.15 ± 1.17) (Table 3). Both groups showed an elevated number of labeled neurons in the area positioned between 7.96 mm and 9.36 mm caudally from bregma. The rostrocaudal distribution and mean values of Fos-IR neurons are shown in figures 7 and 8, respectively. Bright-field photomicrographs of coronal sections of the DR in experimental groups are shown in figures 9-11.

S GROUP				T GROUP		
DR	Mean	SD	SE	Mean	SD	SE
7.16	0.00	0.00	0.00	0.00	0.00	0.00
7.36	0.41	0.00	0.00	0.22	0.00	0.00
7.56	0.84	0.00	0.00	0.41	0.00	0.00
7.76	1.32	0.82	0.33	0.84	1.33	0.44
7.96	2.84	0.82	0.33	3.95	2.07	0.69
8.16	5.13	0.55	0.22	7.10	1.67	0.56
8.36	6.13	1.03	0.42	5.12	1.54	0.51
8.56	7.87	1.10	0.45	6.17	1.50	0.50
8.76	6.31	0.84	0.34	7.71	0.60	0.20
8.96	5.10	0.55	0.22	5.10	0.73	0.24
9.16	5.10	1.47	0.60	5.80	1.45	0.48
9.36	3.60	0.82	0.33	7.13	1.87	0.62
9.56	2.50	1.10	0.45	7.12	2.07	0.69

Table 3. Dorsal raphe nucleus (DR): Distribution of Fos-IR neurons (mean ± SD and SE) in rostrocaudal axis of groups S and T.

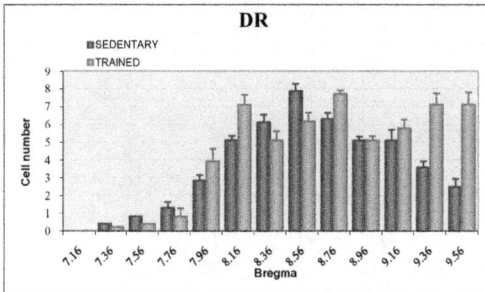

Figure 7. Dorsal raphe nucleus (DR): Distribution of Fos-IR neurons (mean ± SD) in rostrocaudal axis of experimental groups.

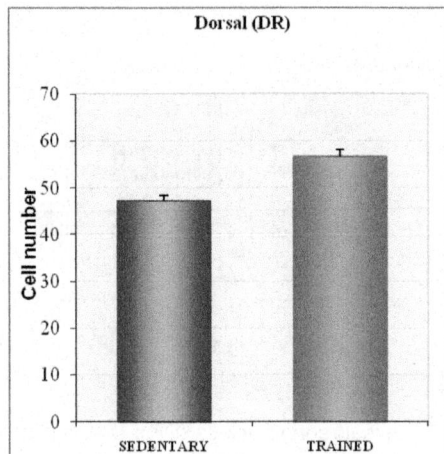

Figure 8. Dorsal raphe nucleus (DR): Total number of Fos-IR neurons (mean ± SD) in experimental groups.

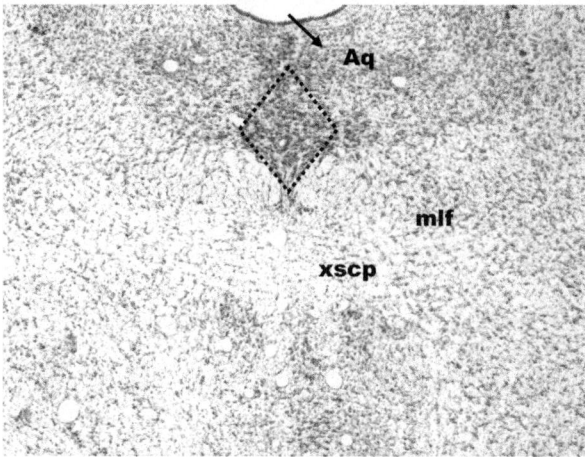

Figure 9. Dorsal raphe nucleus (DR): Bright-field photomicrograph of brain section stained with Nissl method (100x original magnification). Abbreviation: Aq, aqueduct of Sylvius; mlf, medial longitudinal fasciculus; xscp, decussation of the superior cerebellar peduncle.

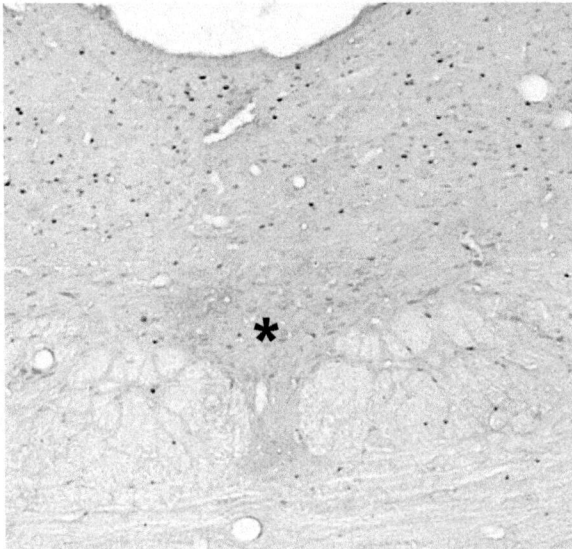

Figure 10. Dorsal raphe nucleus (DR) (*): Bright-field photomicrograph showing Fos-IR neurons in group S animals (100X).

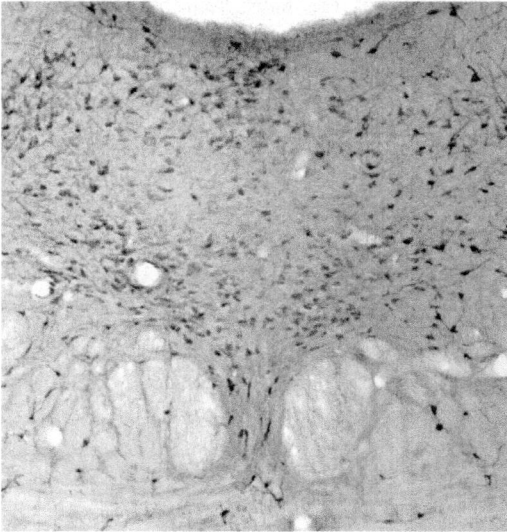

Figure 11. Dorsal raphe nucleus (DR): Bright-field photomicrograph showing Fos-IR neurons in group T animals (100X).

The median raphe nucleus (MnR) showed a greater quantity of Fos-IR neurons in group T (23.89 ± 1.13 Fos-IR neurons, an increase of 12.74%) than in group S (21.19 ± 0.89) (Table 4). In group S, the number of Fos-IR neurons was increased in the areas between levels 7.56mm and 8.16mm, caudally from bregma. This distribution of Fos-IR neurons along the rostrocaudal axis and mean values in the different groups are shown in figures 12 and 13, respectively. Bright-field photomicrographs of the MnR from the experimental groups are shown in figures 14-16.

	S GROUP				T GROUP		
MnR	Mean	SD	SE		Mean	SD	SE
7.36	1.73	0.75	0.31		0.90	0.73	0.24
7.56	4.08	0.75	0.31		3.84	1.12	0.37
7.76	4.88	0.55	0.22		7.71	0.87	0.29
7.96	5.03	0.52	0.21		5.34	0.71	0.24
8.16	5.47	0.98	0.40		6.19	1.17	0.39

Table 4. Median raphe nucleus (MnR): Distribution of Fos-IR neurons (mean ± SD and SE) in rostrocaudal axis of groups S and T.

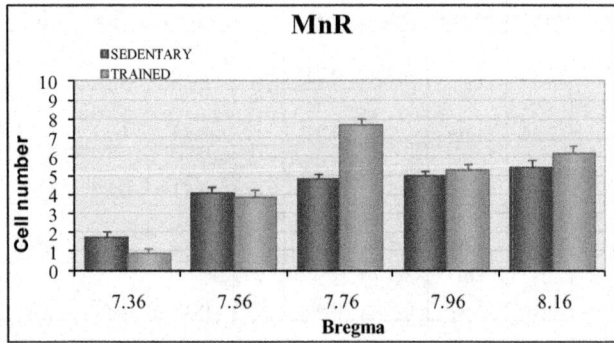

Figure 12. Median raphe nucleus (MnR): Distribution of Fos-IR neurons (mean ± SD) in rostrocaudal axis in the experimental groups

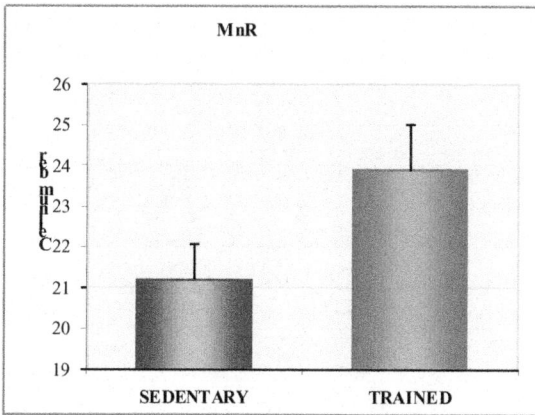

Figure 13. Median raphe nucleus (MnR): Total number of
Fos-IR neurons (mean ± SD) in experimental groups.

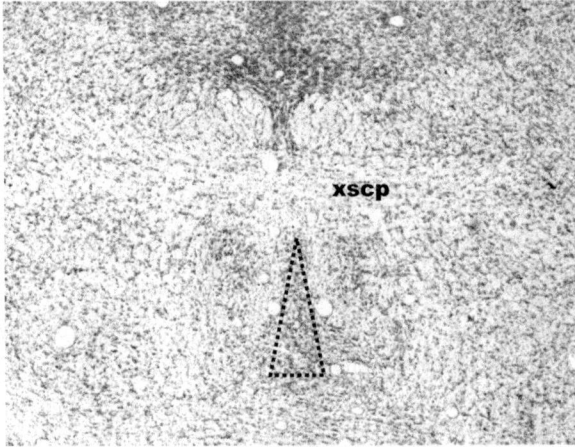

Figure 14. Median raphe nucleus (MnR): Bright-field photomicrography showing Nissl stain (100X).

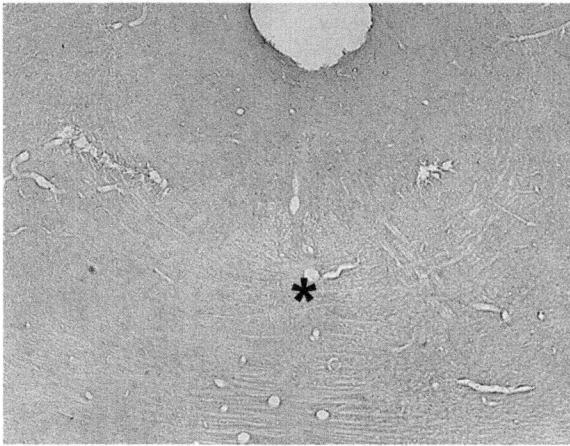

Figure 15. Median raphe nucleus (MnR) (*): Bright-field photomicrography showing Fos-IR neurons in group S animals (100X).

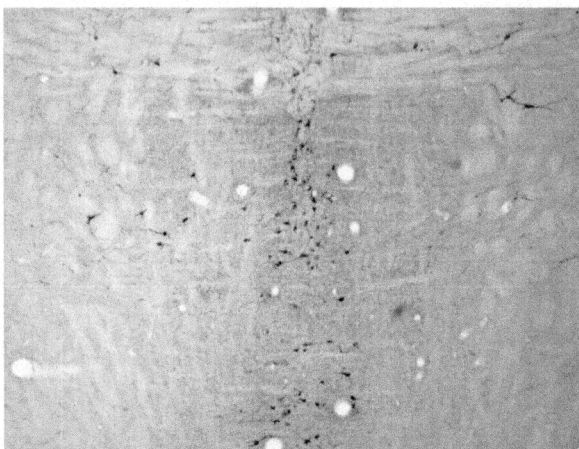

Figure 16. Median raphe nucleus (MnR): Bright-field photomicrography showing Fos-IR neurons in group T animals (100X).

The paramedian raphe nucleus (PMnR) had fewer Fos-IR neurons (4.08 ± 0.44, a decrease of 31.12%) in group T than in group S (5.35 ± 0.44) (Table 5). This was the only raphe nuclei to show greater mean number of Fos-IR neurons in the sedentary group among all studied nuclei. The highest density of Fos-IR neurons was concentrated between 7.76mm and 7.96mm, caudally from bregma. The rostrocaudal distribution of Fos-IR neurons and mean values within experimental groups are shown in figures 17-18 and table 05, respectively. Illustrations and bright-field photomicrographs of the PMnR nucleus in the experimental groups are shown in figures 19-21.

	S GROUP				T GROUP		
PMnR	Mean	SD	SE		Mean	SD	SE
7.56	1.47	0.52	0.21		0.15	0.33	0.11
7.76	1.84	0.63	0.26		1.33	0.67	0.22
7.96	1.33	0.41	0.17		1.66	0.44	0.15
8.16	0.71	0.00	0.00		0.94	0.71	0.24

Table 5. Paramedian raphe nucleus (PMnR): Distribution of Fos-IR neurons (mean ± SD and SE) in rostrocaudal axis of groups S and T.

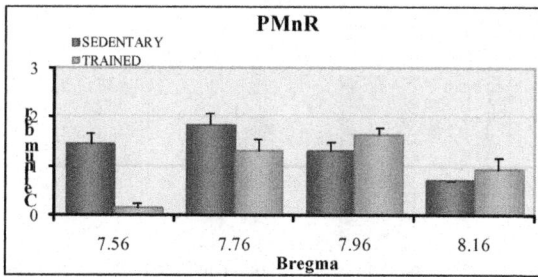

Figure 17. **P**aramedian raphe nucleus (PMnR): Distribution of Fos-IR neurons (mean ± SD) in rostrocaudal axis in the experimental groups.

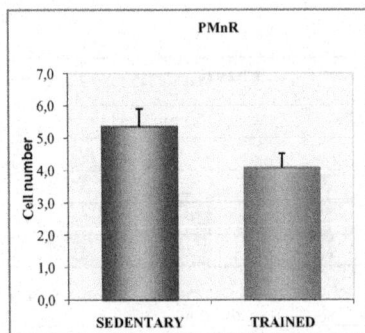

Figure 18. Paramedian raphe nucleus (PMnR): Total number of Fos-IR neurons (mean ± SD) in experimental groups.

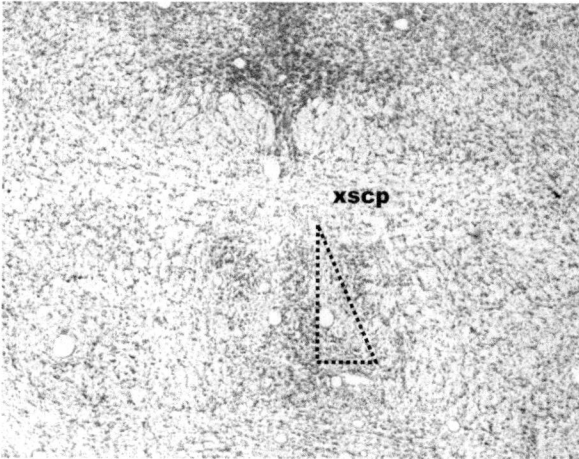

Figure 19. Paramedian raphe nucleus (PMnR): Bright-
field photomicrography showing Nissl stain (100X).

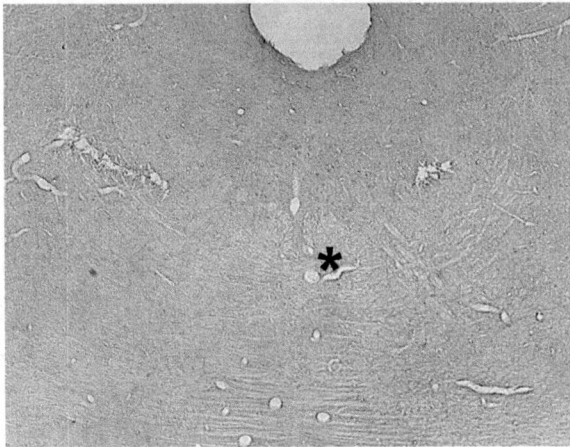

Figure 20. Paramedian raphe nucleus (PMnR) (*): Bright-field photomicrography showing Fos-IR neurons in group S animals (100X).

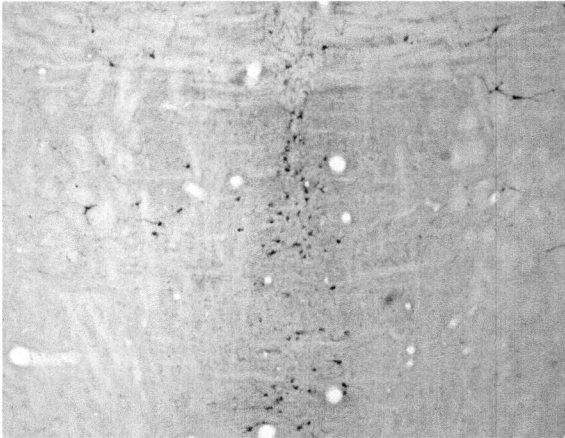

Figure 21. Paramedian raphe nucleus (PMnR): Bright-field photomicrography showing Fos-IR neurons in group T animals (100X).

The pontine raphe nucleus (PnR) had higher values of Fos-IR neurons in group T (20.18 ± 0.67; increase of 43.42%) than in group S (14.07 ± 0.52) (Table 06). The highest density of labeled neurons was situated between 8.96mm and 9.36mm caudally from bregma. The rostrocaudal distribution of Fos-IR neurons in the PnR nucleus and mean values within the experimental groups are shown in figures 22 and 23. Bright-field photomicrographs of the PnR nucleus are shown in figures 24-26.

S GROUP				T GROUP		
PnR	**Mean**	**SD**	**SE**	**Mean**	**SD**	**SE**
8.16	0.00	0.00	0.00	0.00	0.00	0.00
8.36	0.44	0.00	0.00	1.12	0.00	0.00
8.56	0.81	0.00	0.00	0.84	0.71	0.24
8.76	1.42	0.82	0.33	1.33	1.00	0.33
8.96	2.84	0.52	0.21	3.21	1.45	0.48
9.16	3.12	0.75	0.31	5.62	1.09	0.36
9.36	3,12	0.75	0.31	5.62	1.64	0.55
9.56	2.32	0.52	0.21	2.44	1.41	0.47

Table 6. Pontine raphe nucleus (PnR): Distribution of Fos-IR neurons (mean ± SD and SE) in rostrocaudal axis of groups S and T.

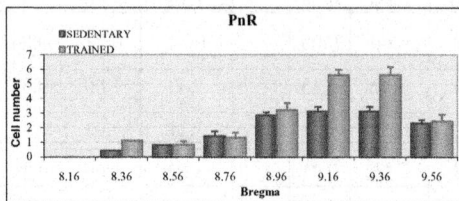

Figure 22. Pontine raphe nucleus (PnR): Distribution of Fos-IR neurons (mean ± SD) in rostrocaudal axis in the experimental groups.

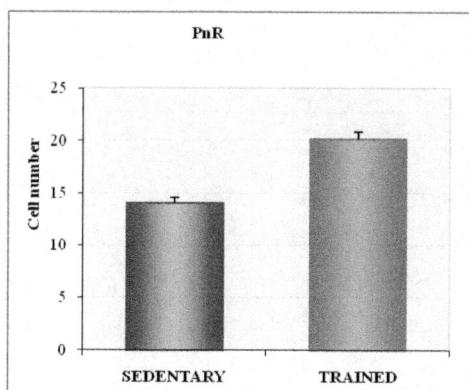

Figure 23. Pontine raphe nucleus (PnR): Total number of Fos-IR neurons (mean ± SD) in experimental groups.

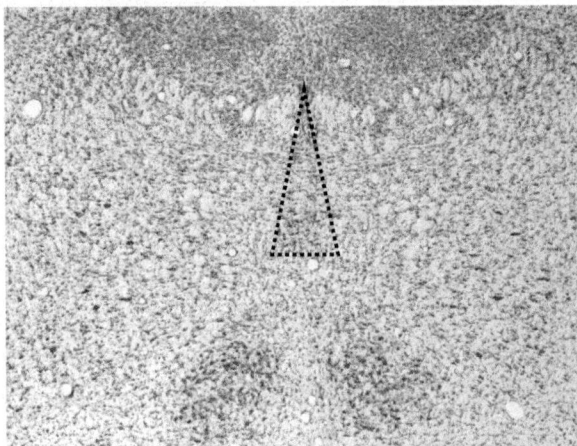

Figure 24. Pontine raphe nucleus (PnR): Bright-field photomicrography showing Nissl stain (100X).

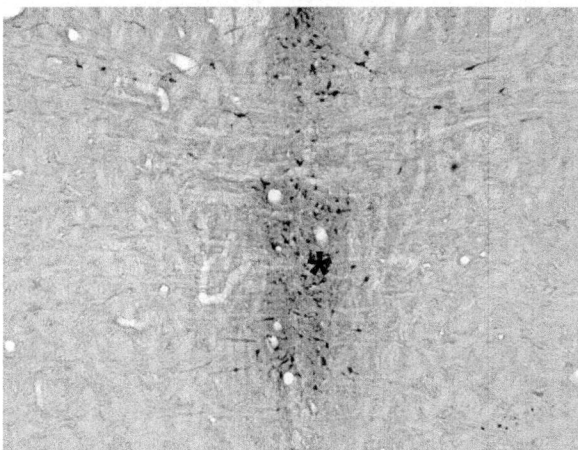

Figure 25. Pontine raphe nucleus (PnR) (*): Bright-field photomicrography showing Fos-IR neurons in group S animals (100X).

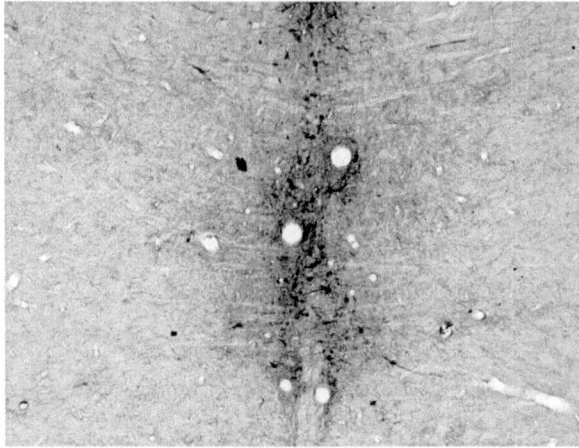

Figure 26. Pontine raphe nucleus (PnR): Bright-field photomicrography showing Fos-IR neurons in group T animals (100X).

The magnus raphe nucleus (RMg) had higher values of Fos-IR neurons in group T (42.68 ± 0.88; an increase of 18.25%) than in group S (36.09 ± 0.89) (Table 7). Most of the labeled neurons were situated between levels 10.56mm and 11.56mm, caudally from bregma. The rostrocaudal distribution of Fos-IR neurons in the PnR nucleus and mean values within the experimental groups are shown in figures 27 and 28. Bright-field photomicrographs of the PnR nucleus in the experimental groups are shown in figures 29-31.

S GROUP				T GROUP		
RMg	Mean	SD	SE	Mean	SD	SE
9.16	0.00	0.00	0.00	0.00	0.00	0.00
9.36	0.00	0.00	0.00	0.00	0.00	0.00
9.56	0.31	0.00	0.00	0.40	0.00	0.00
9.76	0.00	0.00	0.00	0.21	0.00	0.00
9.96	0.39	0.41	0.17	0.71	1.33	0.44
10.16	1.51	0.89	0.37	2.81	2.00	0.67
10.36	4.33	0.55	0.22	4.00	2.05	0.68
10.56	5.38	0.98	0.40	5.81	1.87	0.62
10.76	7.97	1.75	0.71	6.21	1.87	0.62
10.96	4.93	1,03	0.42	6.12	1.59	0.53
11.16	3.80	0.00	0.00	7.33	1.54	0.51
11.36	3.91	0.89	0.37	5.41	2.15	0.72
11.56	1.94	0.84	0.34	2.84	2.40	0.80
11.76	1.62	0.63	0.26	0.83	1.13	0.38

Table 7. Magnus raphe nucleus (RMg): Distribution of Fos-IR neurons (mean ± SD and SE) in rostrocaudal axis of groups S and T.

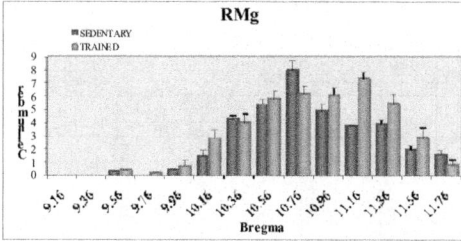

Figure 27. Magnus raphe nucleus (RMg): Distribution of Fos-IR neurons (mean ± SD) in rostrocaudal axis in the experimental groups.

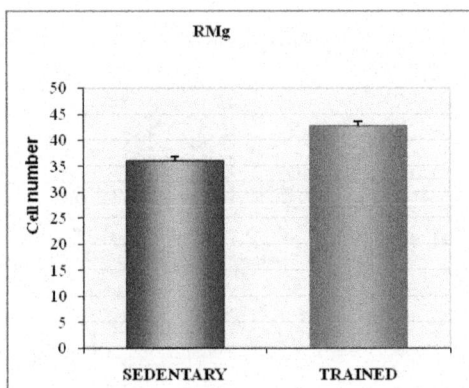

Figure 28. Magnus raphe nucleus (RMg): Total number of Fos-IR neurons (mean ± SD) in experimental groups.

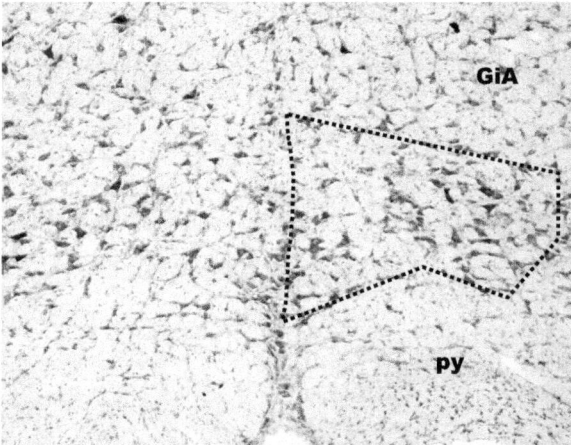

Figure 29. Magnus raphe nucleus (RMg): Bright-field photomicrography showing Nissl stain (100X). Abbreviations: GiA, gigantocellular reticular nucelus, alpha part; py, pyramidal tract.

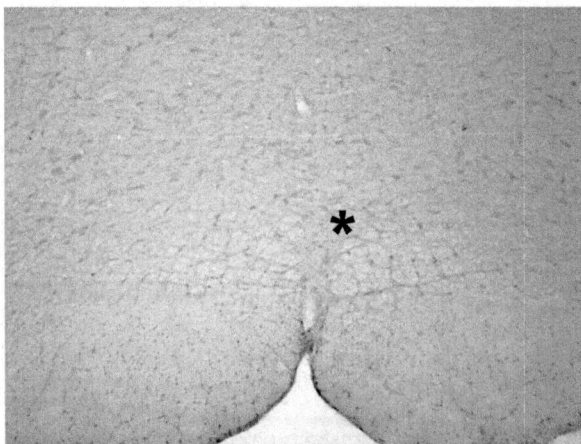

Figure 30. Magnus raphe nucleus (RMg) (*): Bright-field photomicrography showing Fos-IR neurons in group S animals (100X).

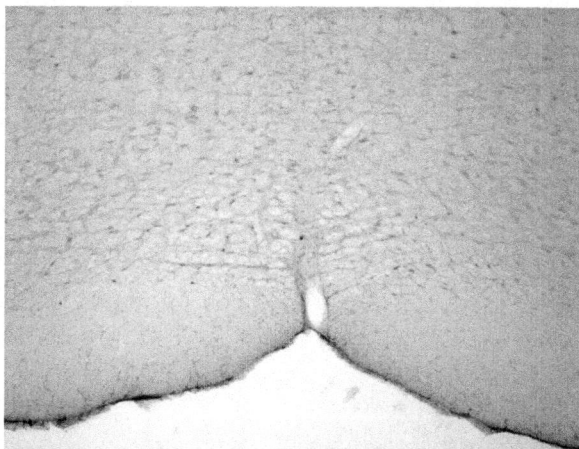

Figure 31. Magnus raphe nucleus (RMg): Bright-field photomicrography showing Fos-IR neurons in group T animals (100X).

The pallidus raphe nucleus (RPa) nucleus had higher values of Fos-IR neurons in group T (57.74 ± 1.13; increase of 30.04%) than in group S (44.40 ± 1.17) (Table 8). The RPa nucleus in group T had the highest labeling density among all raphe nuclei. In both experimental groups, there was a higher density of Fos-IR neurons between levels 11.56 mm and 13.56 mm caudally from bregma. The rostrocaudal distribution of Fos-IR neurons in the RPa nucleus and mean values between the experimental groups are shown in figures 32 and 33. Bright-field photomicrographs of the RPa nucleus in the experimental groups are shown in figures 34-36.

S GROUP				T GROUP		
RPa	Mean	SD	SE	Mean	SD	SE
9.76	0.00	0.00	0.00	0.00	0.00	0.00
9.96	0.00	0.00	0.00	0.00	0.00	0.00
10.16	0.00	0.00	0.00	0.00	0.00	0.00
10.36	0.12	0.00	0.00	0.21	0.00	0.00
10.56	0.12	0.00	0.00	0.21	0.00	0.00
10.76	0.12	0.00	0.00	0.21	0.00	0.00
10.96	0.30	0.00	0.00	0.21	0.00	0.00
11.16	0.50	0.52	0.21	0.41	0.67	0.22
11.36	0.81	0.63	0.26	0.21	0.33	0.11
11.56	1.91	0.75	0.31	0.54	0.50	0.17
11.76	2.83	1.05	0.43	0.54	0.50	0.17
11.96	3.12	1.03	0.42	1.89	1.73	0.58
12.16	4.42	0.75	0.31	4.21	1.00	0.33
12.36	4.42	0.82	0.33	5.21	1.48	0.49
12.56	3.20	0.75	0.31	4.54	0.93	0.31
12.76	5.99	0.75	0.31	6.00	1.48	0.49
12.96	2.47	0.52	0.21	7.31	1.58	0.53
13.16	2.47	0.52	0.21	4.94	1.48	0.49
13.36	2.13	0.82	0.33	5.16	0.87	0.29
13.56	2.81	0.55	0.22	5.00	1.22	0.41
13.76	2.47	0.82	0.33	4.47	1.45	0.48
13.96	1.33	0.82	0.33	4.94	2.24	0.75
14.16	1.53	0.98	0.40	1.12	1.30	0.43
14.36	1.33	0,52	0.21	0.41	0.44	0.15

Table 8. Pallidus raphe nucleus (RPa): Distribution of Fos-IR neurons (mean ± SD and SE) in rostrocaudal axis of groups S and T.

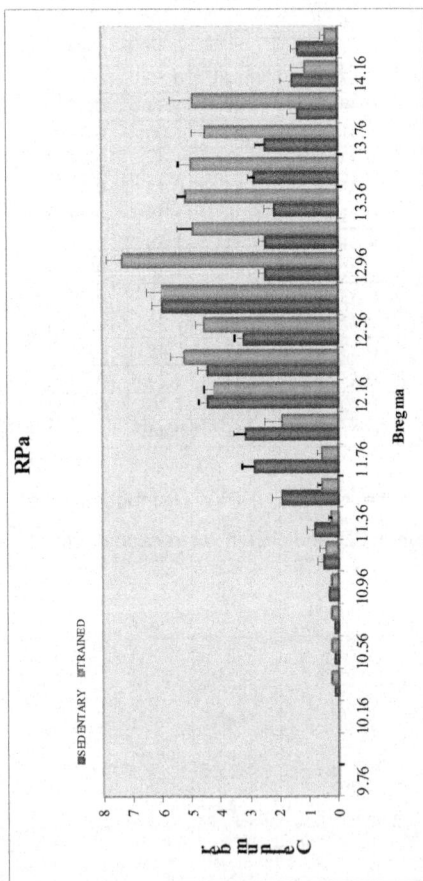

Figure 32. Pallidus raphe nucleus (RPa): Distribution of Fos-IR neurons (mean ± SD) in rostrocaudal axis in the experimental groups.

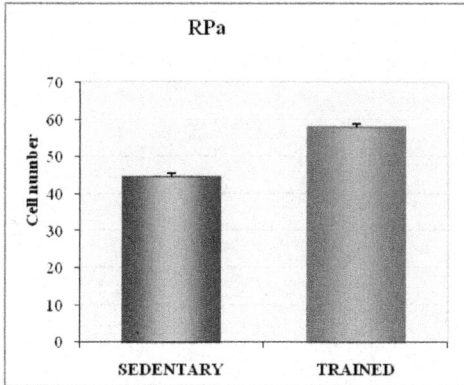

Figure 33. Pallidus raphe nucleus (RPa): Total number of Fos-IR neurons (mean ± SD) in experimental groups.

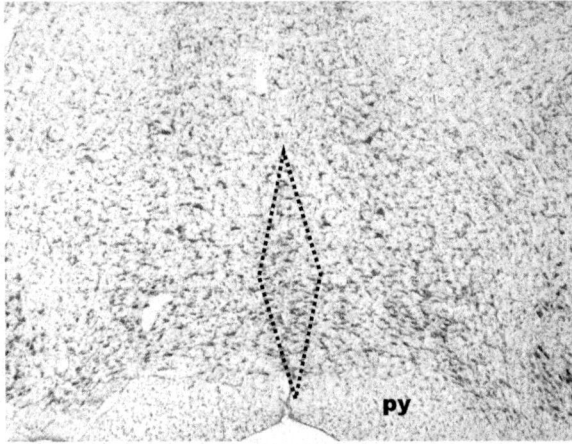

Figure 34. Pallidus raphe nucleus (RPa): Bright-field photomicrography showing Nissl stain (100X). Abbreviations: py, pyramidal tract.

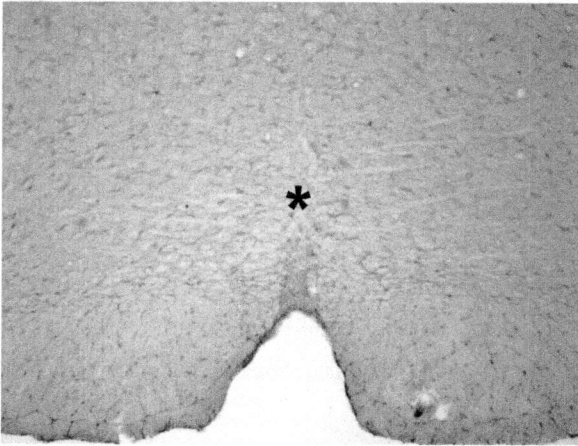

Figure 35. Pallidus raphe nucleus (RPa) (*): Bright-field photomicrography showing Fos-IR neurons in group S animals (100X).

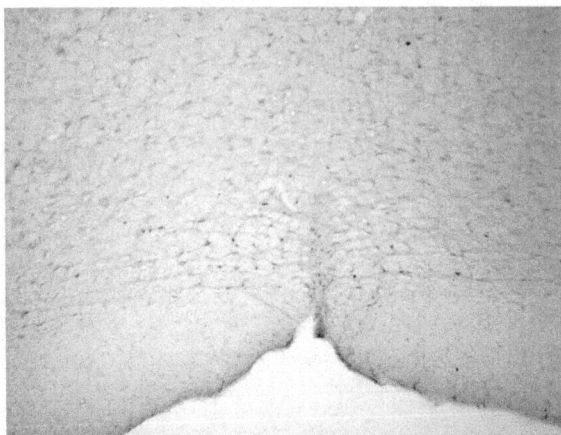

Figure 36. Pallidus raphe nucleus (RPa): Bright-field photomicrography showing Fos-IR neurons in group T animals (100X).

The raphe obscurus nucleus (ROb) showed higher values of Fos-IR neurons in group T (23.98 ± 0.71; increase of 21.72%) than in group S (19.70 ± 0.82) (Table 09). The highest density of labeled cells occurred between levels 12.56 mm and 13.56 mm caudally from bregma. The rostrocaudal distribution of Fos-IR neurons in the ROb nucleus and mean values between experimental groups are shown in figures 37 and 38. Illustrations and bright-field photomicrographs of the ROb nucleus in the experimental groups are shown in figures 39-41.

S GROUP				T GROUP		
ROb	Mean	SD	SE	Mean	SD	SE
11.16	0.00	0.00	0.00	0.00	0.00	0.00
11.36	0.00	0.00	0.00	0.00	0.00	0.00
11.56	0.00	0.00	0.00	0.41	0.00	0.00
11.76	0.21	0.00	0.00	0.21	0.00	0.00
11.96	0.21	0.00	0.00	0.21	0.00	0.00
12.16	0.21	0.00	0.00	0.21	0.00	0.00
12.36	0.54	0.52	0.21	1.21	0.73	0.24
12.56	1.18	0.52	0.21	1.44	1.12	0.37
12.76	1.54	0.41	0.17	3.89	0.87	0.29
12.96	2.36	0.84	0.34	4.33	1.41	0.47
13.16	3.84	0.89	0.37	2.83	1.01	0.34
13.36	3.23	0.41	0.17	1.94	0.88	0.29
13.56	1.94	0.52	0.21	1.88	1.05	0.35
13.76	1.83	0.41	0.17	2.83	1.81	0.60
13.96	1.54	0.52	0.21	1.77	1.05	0.35
14.16	0.86	0.52	0.21	0.41	0.44	0.15
14.36	0.21	0.00	0.00	0.41	0.00	0,00

Table 9. Raphe obscurus nucleus (ROb): Distribution of Fos-IR neurons (mean ± SD and SE) in rostrocaudal axis of groups S and T.

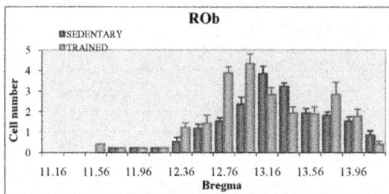

Figure 37. Raphe obscurus nucleus (ROb): Distribution of Fos-IR neurons (mean ± SD) in rostrocaudal axis in the experimental groups

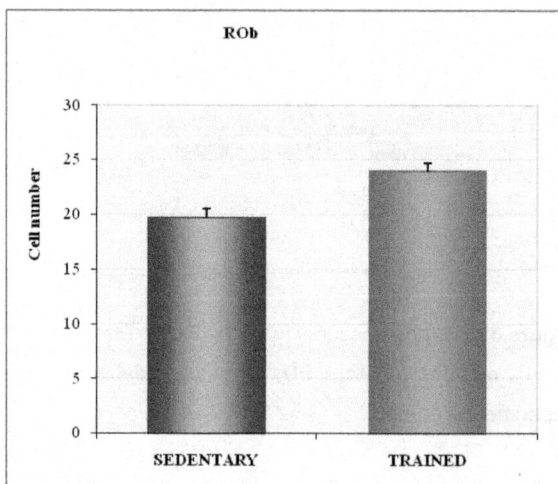

Figure 38. Raphe obscurus nucleus (ROb): Total number of Fos-IR neurons (mean ± SD) in experimental groups.

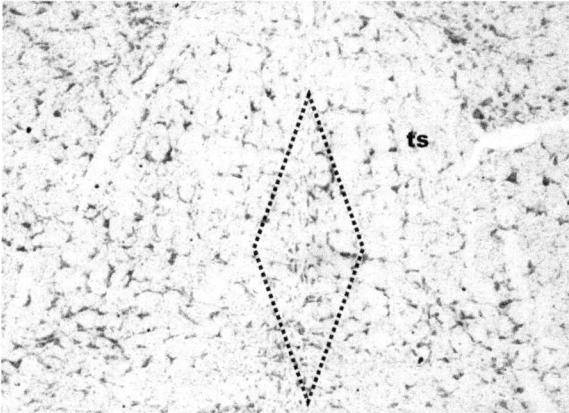

Figure 39. Raphe obscurus nucleus (ROb): Bright-field photomicrography showing Nissl stain (100X). Abbreviation: ts, tectospinal tract.

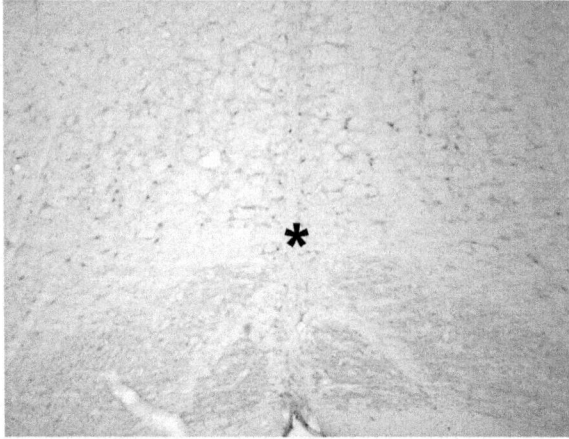

Figure 40. Raphe obscurus nucleus (ROb) (*). Bright-field photomicrography showing Fos-IR neurons in group S animals (100X).

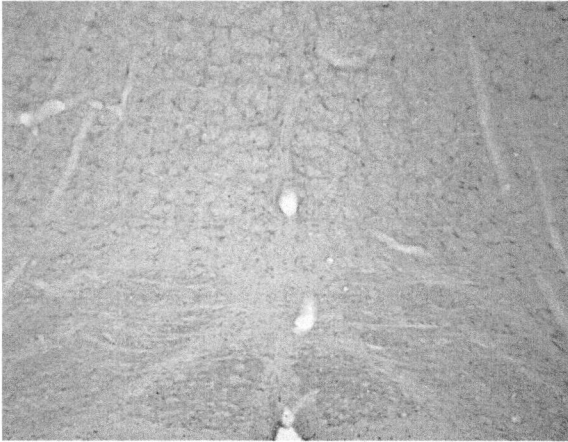

Figure 41. Raphe obscurus nucleus (ROb): Bright-field photomicrography showing Fos-IR neurons in group T animals (100X).

The RPa nucleus showed the highest values of Fos-IR neurons (57.74 in group T and 44.4 in group S), followed by the DR nucleus (56.67 in group T and 47.15 in group S), RMg (42.68 in group T and 36.09 in group S), ROb (23.98 in group T and 19.70 in group S), MnR (23.89 in group T and 21.19 in group S) and PnR (20.18 in group T and 14.07 in group S). In the PMnR nucleus, in contrast to other groups, a higher mean of Fos-IR neurons was observed in group S (5.35 Fos-IR neurons) in relation to group T (4.08). Among all experimental groups, the RPa and DR nuclei showed the highest total absolute values of Fos-IR neurons and the PmR and PnR showed the lowest values, excluding the linear nuclei (Rli and CLi) which showed no Fos-IR neurons in both experimental groups. The absolute values (mean ± SD) of Fos-IR neurons in each raphe nuclei in the different experimental groups are shown in Figure 42.

Briefly, the trained group showed highest density of Fos-IR neurons (variation between 12.74% and 43.42%) in the raphe nuclei, in comparison with the sedentary group. In contrast, the PMnR nucleus showed the highest values of Fos-IR neurons in group S (31.12% higher in relation to group T); however this difference was not statistically significant.

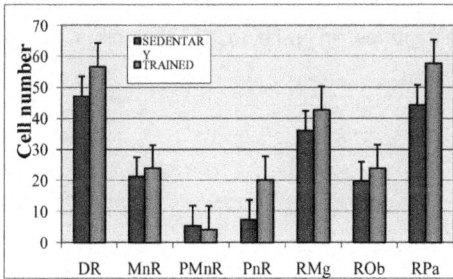

Fig. 42. Distribution of Fos-IR neurons (mean and SD) in different raphe nuclei of experimental groups. Neuron distribution is represented along rostrocaudal axis, where the X axis shows different raphe nuclei and Y axis shows number of labeled cells.

4.3. Statistical Analysis

The analysis of variance (ANOVA) and Tukey´s *post-hoc* test revealed differences among the several nuclei in relation to training. When mean values of several nuclei from the trained group were compared, no significant differences were observed among them.

The PMnR and RPa nuclei showed significant lowest and highest ($p<0.005$) expression of Fos-IR neurons in both experimental groups in relation to the other nuclei, respectively.

5. DISCUSSION

The results of this study demonstrate that moderate swimming induces the production of Fos-protein in neurons located in the raphe nuclei. However, both motor activity and stress may be involved in this physiological stimulation; therefore it is difficult to completely distinguish the effects of both factors.

Previous studies have shown that stress increases (Speciale et al., 1986; Sabol et al., 1990; Hattori et al., 1994; Freed and Yamamoto, 1985) or decreases (Szostak et al., 1986; Schwarting and Huston, 1987; Inoue et al., 1994) brain activity. The basal expression of Fos-protein is extremely low in the raphe nuclei (Morgan and Curran, 1991), which has been evidenced by studies from our laboratory. Thus, a baseline control group was not used in our study.

Chronic activity patterns, as well as prolonged training, may elicit adaptations in both nervous and skeletal-muscular systems (Enoka, 1997). Swimming has been reported as a moderate type of exercise, very similar to typical efforts performed by rats under normal conditions (Ostman-Smith, 1979). In most studies, only male rats were evaluated, since they have no endocrine changes related to the reproductive function, in contrast to hormonal oscillations in female rats that influence the 5-HT central metabolism (Goodman, 1974; Heninger and Charney, 1987).

The raphe nuclei constitute the most prominent source of 5-HT in the CNS. Some studies reported that physical exercise caused an increase in the 5-HT level in the CNS, specifically in the brain stem. This change may be associated with the increase of motor activity and stress when animals are submitted to physical activity for the first time, increasing 5-HT levels by 13% in the brain (Barchas and Freedman, 1963). Physical exercise constitutes a stressor that challenges homeostatic mechanisms. In addition, under certain conditions, such as in anxiety, stress induces an increase of cardio-respiratory and skeletal-muscular activities (Watt and Groove, 1993).

There is a paradigm that physical training elicits similar anatomical and physiological adaptations in different exercises. This was observed in animals submitted to spontaneous exercise in the activity wheel, where stress was markedly reduced (Lambert and Noakes, 1990).

Rats trained according to the moderate intensity swimming protocol showed evident adaptations in the 5-HT metabolism in both brain hemispheres as well as in the brainstem, suggesting that prolonged moderate-intensity exercise activates not only the metabolism but 5-HT synthesis in this region. Moreover, this facilitatory adaptation remains for one week after training (Parnavelas and Papadopolulas, 1989). Similar effects were observed eight weeks after treadmill training (Brown et al., 1979; Dey et al., 1992).

In the present study, the animals were adapted to exercise in the water before training. This procedure consisted of placing animals in temperature controlled water for 30 minutes daily during one week. The animals could reach the bottom of the training tank, so they would not need to exercise. This approach reduced stress contributing to physical training adaptation.

The somatotopic organization of the brain is neuroplastic, insofar that the strength of connections may be altered, for example, during motor learning. This can be observed in studies where the performance of repetitive motor tasks is fundamental for the motor rehabilitation from lesions induced in the primary cortex region which corresponds to the hand and fingers. Thus, the characteristic aspect of voluntary movements improves with practice, as demonstrated by *in vivo* studies observed by MRI analysis (Karni, 1995). This neuroplasticity is potentiated by physical exercise. Experimental studies demonstrated that basal levels of neuromuscular activity are fundamental to maintain normal levels of brain-derived neurotrophic factor (BDNF) (Gomez-Pinilla, 2002).

The effect of weight loss by the reduction of abdominal fat, observed in individuals submitted to prolonged moderate-intensity physical training, parallels a reduction in the risk of diseases and weight re-gain through hypocaloric diets (Mayo *et al.*, 2003). Physical training also promotes glycemic control and decreases arterial blood pressure (Stewart, 2002). Muscle hypertrophy, induced by prolonged physical training, decreases the triglycerides in the blood of men infected by the human immunodeficiency virus (HIV) and treated with antiviral therapy (Yarasheski *et al.*, 2001).

Locomotor activities induce changes in the respiratory and cardiovascular activity in proportion to the performed physical exercise. In hypertensive rats, γ-aminobutyric acid (GABA) -deficiency contributes to raise arterial blood pressure levels, associating a GABAergic function in neuroplasticity control with exercise (Kramer *et al.*, 2002). There are beneficial effects caused by the improvement of cardiovascular health as a result of by physical exercise, promoting changes in central controlling regions of the arterial pressure in hypertensive rats (Kramer *et al.*, 2002). The blood flow increase to the brain when motor cortex areas are involved in a determined behavior indicates that tissue perfusion influences neural activity, which is observed through radioactive xenon injection (Roland *et al.*, 1980).

Immunohistological data demonstrated that physical exercise induces angiogenesis 30 days following the beginning of training, although only in the specific region of the primary motor cortex related to that specific exercise and not in other cortical areas (Swain *et al.*, 2003). Therefore, it can be concluded that the increase in the number of capillaries occurs in several motor areas of the cortex as an adaptation to prolonged motor activity; these changes are chronic and observed even in anesthetized animals when studied by non-invasive techniques (Swain *et al.*, 2003). The PnR is intimately associated with blood vessels, making it permissible to increased f-Trp and Trp uptake during prolonged physical training.

Physical exercises stimulate 5-HT synthesis and central metabolism, as they increase the level of f-Trp and BCAAs, mainly after prolonged exercise sessions (Nybo, 2003; Soares *et al.*, 2003). The increase of the 5-HT precursor amino acid favors the transportation of Trp to the brain and consequently, increases 5-HT synthesis and release (Blomstrand, 2001). Rats trained for 11 weeks exhibited a significant increase in 5-HT (14%) and 5-HIAA (44%) in the brainstem (Blomstrand *et al.*, 1989).

The individual Fos-IR neuron counting carried out in each raphe nucleus, using serial sections showed results in accordance with the literature. Data obtained in this study provide pioneer distinction of the individualized participation of the raphe nuclei in homeostatic responses of young male rats submitted to prolonged physical exercise by immunohistochemistry techniques.

This study provides insights into future approaches on this topic for investigations using neuronal tracers to elucidate afferent and efferent connections of the raphe nuclei associated with prolonged physical training.

6. CONCLUSIONS

1- Trained animals showed behavioral and physiological adaptation to the moderate swimming protocol, due to less effort taken for each training session, validating the model used in the present study,

2- Physical exercise induced differential expression of Fos protein in the various raphe nuclei associated with motricity in both trained and sedentary rats,

3- The Rli and Cli nuclei showed no expression of Fos protein in both groups and,

4- This study distinguished for the first time the individual participation of the various raphe nuclei when comparing sedentary and trained rats, opening perspectives for new approaches on this topic.

7. REFERENCES

1. AGHAJANIAN GK. Modulation of a transient outward current in serotonergic neurones by alpha 1-adrenoceptors. *Nature,* 315: 501-3, 1985.

2. AMERICAN COLLEGE OF SPORTS MEDICINE. The recommended quantity and quality of exercise for developing and maintaining fitness in healthy adults, *Med Sci Sports,* 10: VII-X, 1978.

3. AMERICAN HEART ASSOCIATION. Statement on exercise: benefits and recommendations for physical activity programs for all Americans. *Circulation,* 94: 857-862, 1996.

4. ASMUSSEN E, MAZIN B. A central nervous component in local muscular fatigue. *Eur J Appl Physio Occup Physiol,* 38: 9-15, 1978.

5. BAKER KG, HALLIDAY GM, TÖRK I. Cytoarchitecture of the human dorsal raphe nucleus. *J Comp Neurol,* 301: 147-61,1990.

6. BAKER KG, HALLIDAY GM. Ascending noradrenergic and serotoninergic systems in the human brainstem. Neurotransmitters in the human brain. Tracey DJ (ed.) New York: Plenum Press, 1995.

7. BARCHAS JD, FREEDMAN DX. Brain amines: response to physiological stress. *Biochem Pharmacol,* 12: 1232-5, 1963.

8. BASSIT RA, SAWADA LA, BACURAU RF, NAVARRO F, COSTA ROSA LF. The effect of BCAA supplementation upon the immune response of triathletes. *Med Sci Sports Exerc,* 32: 1214-9, 2000.

9. BÉLANGER M, DREW T, ROSSIGNOL S. Spinal locomotion: a comparison of the kinematics and the

electromyographic activity in the same animal before and after spinalization. *Acta Biol Hung*, 39: 151-4, 1988.

10. BJÖRKLUND A, FALCK B, STENEVI U. Classification of monoamine neurones in the rat mesencephalon: distribution of a new monoamine neurone system. *Brain Res*, 32: 269-85, 1971.

11. BLAIR SN, GOODYEAR NN, GIBBONS LW, COOPER KW. Physical fitness and incidence of hypertension in healthy normotensive men and women. *JAMA*, 252: 487-90, 1984.

12. BLANKS RH. Afferents to cerebellar flocculus in cat with special reference to pathways conveying vestibular, visual (optokinetic) and oculomotor signals. *J Neurocytol*, 19: 628-42, 1990.

13. BLOMSTRAND E, PERRETT D, PARRY-BILLINGS M, NEWSHOLME EA. Effect of sustained exercise on plasma amino acid concentrations and on 5-hydroxytryptamine metabolism in six different brain regions in the rat. *Acta Physiol Scand*, 136: 473-81, 1989.

14. BLOMSTRAND E. Amino acids and central fatigue. *Amino Acids*, 20: 25-34, 2001.

15. BOWKER RM. The relationship between descending serotonin projections and ascending projections in the nucleus raphe magnus: a double labeling study. *Neurosci Lett*, 70: 348-53,1986.

16. BRINES R, HOFFMAN-GOETZ L, PEDERSEN BK. Can you exercise to make your immune system fitter? *Immunol today*, 17: 252-4, 1996.

17. BRODAL A. The reticular formation and some related nuclei. In: Neurological anatomy in relation to clinical medicine. 3rd ed. New York: Oxford University Press, pp. 394-447, 1981.

18. BROWN BS, PAYNE T, KIM C, MOORE G, KREBS P, MARTIN W. Chronic responses of rat brain norepinephrine

and serotonin levels to endurance training. *J Appl Physiol*, 46: 19-23, 1979.

19. CALABRESE RL. Cellular, synaptic, network, and modulatory mechanisms involved in rhythm generation. *Curr Opin Neurobiol*, 8: 710-7, 1998.

20. CARPENTER MB. Core text of Neuroanatomy. 4th ed. Baltimore: Willians & Wilkins, 1991.

21. CHEN L, GLOVER JN, HOGAN PG, RAO A, HARRISON SC. Structure of the DNA-binding domains from NFAT, Fos and Jun bound specifically to DNA. *Nature*, 392: 42-8, 1998.

22. CIRELLI CE, TONONI G. On the functional significance of c-fos induction during the sleep-waking cycle. *Sleep*, 23: 453-69, 2000.

23. COSTILL DL, THOMAS R, ROBERGS RA, PASCOE D, LAMBERT C, BARR S, FINK WJ. Adaptations to swimming training: influence of training volume. *Med Sci Sports Exerc*, 23: 371-7, 1991.

24. COYLE EF. Integration of the physiological factors determining endurance performance ability. *Exercise and sport Sciences Reviews*, vol 23. Baltimore: Williams & Wilkins, pp. 25-63, 1995.

25. CURRAN T, TEICH NM. Candidate product of the FBJ murine osteosarcoma virus oncogene: Characterization of a 55.000-dalton phosphoprotein. *J Virol*, 42: 114-22, 1982.

26. DAHLSTRÖM A, FUXE K. Localization of monoamines in the lower brain stem. *Experientia*, 20: 398-9, 1964.

27. DANIELS J, FITTS R, SHEEHAN G. *Conditioning for Distance Running – scientific aspects*. New York: John Wiley & Son, 1978.

28. DEY S, SINGH RH, DEY PK. Exercise training: significance of regional alterations in serotonin metabolism

of the rat brain in relation to antidepressant effect of exercise. *Physiol Behav,* 52: 1095-9, 1992.

29. DINARDO LA, TRAVERS JB. Distribution of fos-like immunoreactivity in the medullary reticular formation of the rat after gustatory elicited ingestion and rejection behaviors. *J Neurosci,* 17: 3826-39, 1997.

30. DISHMAN RK. Compliance/adherence in health-related exercise. *Health Psychol,* 1: 237-67, 1982.

31. DISHMAN RK. Physical activity and mental health. In: Friedman H (Ed.). Encyclopedia of Mental Health. Orlando: Academic Press. Vol 3, pp. 171-88, 1998.

32. DISHMAN RK. The impact of behavior on quality of life. *Qual Life Res,* 12: 43-9, 2003.

33. DRAISCI G, IADAROLA MJ. Temporal analysis of increases in c-fos, preprodynorphin and preproenkephalin mRNAs in rat spinal cord. *Brain Res Mol Brain Res,* 6: 31-7, 1989.

34. DWYER D, BROWNING J. Endurance training in Wistar rats decreases receptor sensitivity to a serotonin agonist. *Acta Physiol Scand,* 170: 211-6, 2000.

35. ENOKA RM. Neural adaptations with chronic physical activity. *J Biomech,* 30: 447-55, 1997.

36. FOO H, MASON P. Brainstem modulation of pain during sleep and waking. *Sleep Med Rev,* 7:145-54, 2003.

37. FOX EL, BARTELS R, BILLINGS CE, O'BRIEN R, BASON R, MATHEWS DK. Frequency and duration of interval training programs and changes in aerobic power. *J Appl Physiol,* 38: 481-4, 1975.

38. FOX EL, BARTELS RL, BILLINGS CE, MATHEWS DK, BASON R, WEBB WM. Intensity and distance on interval training programs and changes in aerobic power. *Med Sci Sports,* 5: 18-22, 1973.

39. FREED CR, YAMAMOTO BK. Regional brain dopamine metabolism: a marker for the speed, direction and posture of moving animals. *Science,* 229: 62-5, 1985.

40. GANDEVIA SC, ALLEN GM, MCKENZIE DK. Central fatigue. Critical issues, quantification and practical implications. *Adv Exp Med Biol,* 384: 281-94, 1995.

41. GETTMAN LR, POLLOCK ML, DURSTINE JL, WARD A, AYRES J, LINNERUD AC. Physiological responses of men to 1, 3 and 5 day per week training programs. *Res Q.* 47: 638-46, 1976.

42. GETTMAN LR. Economic benefits of physical activity. *Physical Fitness and Sports Research Digest.* 2: 1-6, 1996.

43. RIBOTTA M, PROVENCHER J, FERABOLI-LOHNHERR D, ROSSIGNOL S, PRIVAT AE, ORSAL D. Activation of locomotion in adult chronic spinal rats is achieved by transplantation of embryonic raphe cells reinnervating a precise lumbar level. *J Neurosci,* 20: 5144-52, 2000.

44. GOLDSPINK G. Malleability of the motor system: a comparative approach. *J Exp Biol,* 115: 375-91, 1985.

45. GOLLNICK PD, TIMSON BF, MOORE RL, RIEDY M. Muscular enlargement and numbers of fibers in skeletal muscles of rats. *J Appl Physiol,* 50: 936-43, 1981.

46. GÓMEZ-PINILLA F, YING Z, ROY RR, MOLTENI R, EDGERTON VR. Voluntary exercise induces a BDNF-mediated mechanism that promotes neuroplasticity. *J Neurophysiol,* 88: 2187-95, 2002.

47. GOODMAN HM. In: Mountcastle VD (Ed.). Reproduction in Medical Physiology. St Louis: Mosby. Vol. 13, pp. 1741-75, 1974.

48. GORDON T, PATTULLO MC. Plasticity of muscle fiber and motor unit types. *Exerc Sports Sci Rev,* 21: 331-62, 1993.

49. GRILLNER S. Control of locomotion in bipeds, tetrapods and fish. In: Brooks V (Ed.). Handbook of Physiology. The Nervous system II. Bethesda: American Physiological Society, pp 1179-1236, 1981.

50. HALBERSTADT AL, BALABAN CD. Organization of projections from the raphe nuclei to the vestibular nuclei in rats. Neuroscience, 120: 573-94, 2003.

51. HATTORI S, NAOI M, NISHINO H. Striatal dopamine turnover during treadmill running in the rat: relation to the speed of running. Brain Res Bull, 35: 41-9, 1994.

52. HAY-SCHMIDT A, VRANG N, LARSEN PJ, MIKKELSEN JD. Projections from the raphe nuclei to the suprachiasmatic nucleus of the rat. J Chem Neuroanat, 25: 293-310, 2003.

53. HELMRICH SP, RAGLAND DR, LEUNG RW, PAFFENBARGER RS Jr. Physical activity and reduced occurrence of non-insulin-dependent diabetes mellitus. N Engl J Med, 325: 147-52, 1991.

54. HENINGER GR, CHARNEY DS. Mechanism of action of antidepressant treatments: Implications for the etiology and treatment of depressive disorders. In: Meltzer HY (Ed.). Psychopharmacology: The third generation of progress. New York: Raven Press, pp. 535-544, 1987.

55. HOFFMAN GE, LYO D. Anatomical markers of activity in neuroendocrine systems: are we all 'Fos-ed out'? J Neuroendocrinol, 14: 259-68, 2002.

56. HOLSTEGE G, KUYPERS HG. The anatomy of brain stem pathways to the spinal cord in cat. A labeled amino acid tracing study. Prog Brain Res, 57: 145-75, 1982.

57. HOLSTEGE G. The basic, somatic and emotional components of the motor system in mammals. In: Paxinos G (Ed.).The Rat Nervous System, 2nd ed. San Diego: Academic Press, pp. 137-154, 1995.

58. HOLSTEGE JC, KYUPERS HG. Brainstem projections to spinal motoneurons: an update. *Neuroscience,* 23: 809-21, 1987.

59. HONRADO GI, JOHNSON RS, GOLOMBEK DA, SPIEGELMAN BM, PAPAIOANNOU VE, RALPH MR. The circadian system of c-fos deficient mice. *J Comp Physiol A,* 178: 563-70,1996.

60. INOUE T, TSUCHIYA K, KOYAMA T. Regional changes in dopamine and serotonin activation with various intensity of physical and physichological stress in the rat brain. *Pharmacol Biochem Behav,* 49: 911-20, 1994.

61. JACKSON JH, SHARKEY BJ, JOHNSTON LP. Cardiorespiratory adaptations to training and specified frequencies. *Res Q,* 39: 295-300, 1968.

62. JACOBS BL, AZMITIA EC. Structure and function of the brain serotonin system. *Physiol Rev,* 72: 165-229, 1992.

63. JACOBS BL, FORNAL CA. 5-HT and motor control: a hypothesis. *Trends Neurosci,* 16: 346-52, 1993.

64. JONES AM, CARTER H. The effect of endurance training on parameters of aerobic fitness. *Sports Med,* 29: 373-86, 2000.

65. KAEHLER ST, SINGEWALD N, SINNER C, THURNHER C, PHILIPPU A. Conditioned fear and inescapable shock modify the release of serotonin in the locus coeruleus. *Brain Res,* 859: 249-54, 2000.

66. KALASKA JF, CRAMMOND DJ. Cerebral cortical mechanisms of reaching movements. *Science,* 255: 1517-23, 1992.

67. KANDEL ER, SCHWARTZ JH, JESSELL TM. Principles of neural science. 4th ed. New York: Mcgraw-Hill, 2000.

68. KARNI A, MEYER G, JEZZARD P, ADAMS MM, TURNER R, UNGERLEIDER LG. Functional MRI

evidence for adult motor cortex plasticity during motor skill learning. *Nature,* 377: 155-8, 1995.

69. KIEHN O, HOUNSGAARD J, SILLAR KT. Basic building blocks of vertebrate spinal central pattern generators. In: Stein PSG, Selverston AI and Stuart DG (Ed.) Neurons, Networks and Motor Behavior. Cambridge: MIT Press, pp. 47-59. 1997.

70. KNUTTGEN HG, NORDESJÖ LO, OLLANDER B, SALTIN B. Physical conditioning through interval training with young male adults. *Med Sci Sports,* 5: 220-6, 1973.

71. KOHL HW, GORDON NF, VILLEGAS JA, BLAIR SN. Cardiorespiratory fitness, glycemic status, and mortality risk in men. *Diabetes Care,* 15: 184-92, 1992.

72. KRAMER JM, BEATTY JA, PLOWEY ED, WALDROP TG. Exercise and hypertension: a model for central neural plasticity. *Clin Exp Pharmacol Physiol,* 29: 122-6, 2002.

73. KRUKOFF TL. Expression of c-fos in studies of central autonomic and sensory systems. *Mol Neurobiol,* 7: 247-63, 1993.

74. LAMBERT MI, NOAKES TD. Spontaneous running increases VO_{2max} and running performance in rats. *J Appl Physiol,* 68: 400-3, 1990.

75. LANCHA JÚNIOR AH, SANTOS MF, PALANCH AC, CURI R. Supplementation of aspartate, asparagine and carnitine in the diet causes marked changes in the ultrastructure of soleus muscle. *J Submicrosc Cytol Pathol,* 29: 405-8, 1997.

76. LAUDANNA A, NOGUEIRA MI, MARIANO M. Expression of Fos protein in the rat central nervous system in response to noxious stimulation: effects of chronic inflammation of the superior cervical ganglion. *Braz J Med Biol Res,* 31: 847-50, 1998.

77. LE BIHAN D, KARNI A. Applications of magnetic resonance imaging to the study of human brain function. *Curr Opin Neurobiol,* 5:231-7, 1995.

78. LEE IM. Physical activity and Cancer. *Physical Activity and Fitness Research Digest,* 2: 1-8, 1995.

79. LEVITT P, RAKIC P, GOLDMAN-RAKIC PS. Comparative assessment of monoamine afferents in mammalian cerebral cortex. In: Descarries L, Reader T and Jasper HH (Ed.). Monoamine innervations of cerebral cortex. New York: Alan R. Liss, pp. 41-59, 1984.

80. LISTE I, GUERRA MJ, CARUNCHO HJ, LABANDEIRA-GARCIA JL. Treadmill running induces striatal Fos expression via NMDA glutamate and dopamine receptors. *Exp Brain Res,* 115: 458-69, 1997.

81. MACKINNON LT. Chronic exercise training effects on immune function. *Med Sci Sports Exerc,* 32: S539-76, 2000.

82. DAVIS JM, ALDERSON NL, WELSH RS. Serotonin and central nervous system fatigue: nutritional considerations. *Am J Clin Nutr,* 72: 573S-8, 2000.

83. MARTINS E Jr, LIGEIRO de OLIVEIRA AP, FIALHO de ARAUJO AM, TAVARES de LIMA W, CIPOLLA-NETO J, COSTA ROSA LF. Melatonin modulates allergic lung inflammation. *J Pineal Res,* 31: 363-9, 2001.

84. MARTINS RA, CUNHA MR, NEVES AP, MARTINS M, TEIXEIRA-VERÍSSIMO M, TEIXEIRA AM. Effects of aerobic conditioning on salivary IgA and plasma IgA, IgG and IgM in older men and women. *Int J Sports Med,* 30: 906-12, 2009.

85. MITTLEMAN MA, MACLURE M, TOFLER GH, SHERWOOD JB, GOLDBERG RJ, MULLER JE. Triggering of acute myocardial infarction by heavy physical exertion. Protection against triggering by regular exertion.

determinants of myocardial infarction onset study investigators. *N Engl J Med,* 329: 1677-83, 1993.

86. MAYO MJ, GRANTHAM JR, BALASEKARAN G. Exercise-induced weight loss preferentially reduces abdominal fat. *Med Sci Sports Exerc,* 35: 207-13, 2003.

87. MEEUSEN R, DE MEIRLEIR K. Exercise and brain neurotransmission. *Sports Med,* 20: 160-88, 1995.

88. MILLER RG, KENT-BRAUN JA, SHARMA KR, WEINER MW. Mechanisms of human muscle fatigue. Quantitating the contribution of metabolic factors and activation impairment. *Adv Exp Med Biol,* 384: 195-210, 1995.

89. MORGAN JI, CURRAN T. Stimulus-transcription coupling in the nervous system: involvement of the inducible proto-oncogenes fos and jun. *Annu Rev Neurosci,* 14: 421-51, 1991.

90. MORGAN JI. CURRAN T. Stimulus-transcription coupling in neurons: role of cellular immediate-early genes. *Trends Neurosci,* 12: 459-62, 1989.

91. MORRISON JH, GRZANNA R, MOLLIVER ME, COYLE JT. The distribution and orientation of noradrenergic fibers in neocortex of the rat: an immunofluorescence study. *J Comp Neurol,* 181: 17-39, 1978.

92. MOSTARDI R, GANDEE R, CAMPBELL T. Multiple daily training and improvement in aerobic power. *Med Sci Sports,* 7: 82, 1975.

93. MUNSAT TL, MCNEAL D, WATERS R. Effects of nerve stimulation on human muscle. *Arch Neurol,* 33: 608-17, 1976.

94. NEWSHOLME EA, ACWORTH IN, BLOMSTRAND E. Aminoacids brain neurotransmitters and a functional link between muscle and brain that is important in sustained

exercise. In: Benzi G (Ed.). Advances in myochemistry. London: John Libbey Eurotext, pp. 127-33, 1987.

95. NEWSHOLME EA, BLOMSTRAND E. The plasma level of some amino acids and physical and mental fatigue. *Experientia,* 52: 413-5, 1996.

96. NIELSEN B, NYBO L. Cerebral changes during exercise in the heat. *Sports Med,* 33: 1-11, 2003.

97. NIH Consensus Development Panel on Physical activity and Cardiovascular Health, Physical activity and cardiovascular health. *JAMA,* 276:241-6, 1995.

98. NOAKES TD. Physiological models to understand exercise fatigue and the adaptations that predict or enhance athletic performance. *Scand J Med Sci Sports,* 10: 123-45, 2000.

99. NYBO L. CNS fatigue and prolonged exercise: effect of glucose supplementation. *Med Sci Sports Exerc,* 34: 589-94, 2003.

100. OSTMAN-SMITH I. Adaptive changes in the sympathetic nervous system and some effector organs of the rat following long term exercise or cold acclimation and the role of cardiac sympathetic nerves in the genesis of compensatory cardiac hyperthrophy. *Acta Physiol Scand,* 477:1-118, 1979.

101. PARENT A. Identification of the pallidal and peripallidal cells projecting to the habenula in monkey. *Neurosci Lett,* 15: 159-64, 1979.

102. PARK HJ, LEE YL, KWON HY, SUH SW, YON JH. Pancreatic exocrine secretion in response to median raphe stimulation in anesthetized rats. *Pancreas,* 10: 407-12, 1995.

103. PARNAVELAS JG, PAPADOPOULOS GC. The monoaminergic innervations of the cerebral cortex is not diffuse and nonspecific. *Trends Neurosci,* 12: 315-9, 1989.

104.   PATE RR, BRANCH JD. Training for endurance sport. *Med Sci Sports Exerc,* 24: S340-3, 1992.

105.   PATE RR, PRATT M, BLAIR SN, HASKELL WL, MACERA CA, BOUCHARD C, BUCHNER D, ETTINGER W, HEATH GW, KING AC, KRISKA A, LEON AS, MARCUS BH, MORRIS J, PAFFENBARGER RS, PATRICK K, POLLACK ML, RIPPE JM, SALLIS J, WILMORE JH . Physical activity and public health: A recommendation from the Centers for Disea se Control and Prevention and the American College of Sports Medicine. *JAMA,* 273: 402-7, 1995.

106.   PAULUS MP, GEYER MA. Three independent factors characterize spontaneous rat motor activity. *Behav Brain Res,* 53: 11-20, 1993.

107.   PAUVERT V, PIERROT-DESEILLIGNY E, ROTHWELL JC. Role of spinal premotoneurones in mediating corticospinal input to forearm motoneurones in man. *J Physiol,* 508: 301-12, 1998.

108.   PAXINOS G, WATSON C. The Rat Brain in Stereotaxic Coordinates. 4th ed. San Diego: Academic Press, 1998.

109.   PEDERSEN BK. Chronic exercise and the immune system. In: Pedersen BK (Ed.). Exercise immunology. Chapter 7. New York: Chapman and Hall, pp.113-141, 1997.

110.   POLLOCK CM, SCHADWICK RE. Allometry of muscle, tendon, and elastic energy storage capacity in mammals. *Am J Physiol,* 266: R1022-31, 1994.

111.   POLLOCK M, CURETON T, GRENINGER L. Effects of frequency of training on working capacity, cardiovascular function and body composition on adult men. *Med Sci Sports,* 1: 70-4, 1969.

112.   PROCHASKA JO, DICLEMENTE CC. Stages and processes of self-change on smoking: toward an

integrative model of change. *J Consult Clin Psychol,* 51: 390-5, 1983.

113.   RAMÓN-MOLINER E, NAUTA WJ. The isodendritic core of the brain stem. *J Comp Neurol,* 126: 311-35, 1966.

114.   RASMUSSEN K, GLENNON RA, AGHAJANIAN GK. Phenethylamine hallucinogens in the locus coeruleus: potency of action correlates with rank order of 5-HT2 binding affinity. *Eur J Pharmacol,* 132: 79-82, 1986.

115.   RAVEN PB, SQUIRES WG. What is science? *Med Sci Sports Exerc,* 21: 351-2, 1989.

116.   RIBEIRO-DO-VALLE LE. Serotoninergic neurons in the caudal raphe nuclei discharge in association with activity of masticatory muscles. *Braz J Med Biol Res,* 30: 79-83, 1997.

117.   ROCHE M, COMMONS KG, PEOPLES A, VALENTINO RJ. Circuitry underlying regulation of the serotonergic system by swim stress. *J Neurosci,* 23: 970-7, 2003.

118.   ROLAND PE, LARSEN B, LASSEN NA, SKINHØJ E. Supplementary motor area and others cortical areas in organization of voluntary movements in man. *J Neurophysiol,* 43: 118-36, 1980.

119.   ROWLAND NE, FREGLY MJ, HAN L, SMITH G. Expression of Fos in rat brain in relation to sodium appetite: furosemide and cerebroventricular renin. *Brain Res,* 728: 90-6, 1996.

120.   SABOL KE, RICHARDS JB, FREED CR. In vivo dialysis measurements of dopamine and DOPAC in rats trained to turn on a circular treadmill. *Pharmacol Biochem Behav,* 36: 21-8, 1990.

121.   SCHWARTING R, HUSTON JP. Dopamine and serotonin metabolism in brain sites ipsi- and contralateral

to direction of conditioned turning in rats. *J Neurochem,* 48: 1473-9, 1987.

122.   SMITH DA, FLYNN JP. Afferent projections to quiet attack sites in cat hypothalamus. *Brain Res,* 194: 29-40, 1980.

123.   SMITH KJ, HALL SM. Nerve conduction during peripheral demyelination and remyelination. *J Neurol Sci,* 48: 201-19, 1980.

124.   SOARES DD, LIMA NR, COIMBRA CC, MARUBAYASHI U. Evidence that tryptophan reduces mechanical efficiency and running performance in rats. *Pharmacol Biochem Behav,* 74: 357-62, 2003.

125.   SPECIALE SG, MILLER JD, McMILLEN BA, GERMAN DC. Activation of specific central dopamine pathways: locomotion and footshock. *Brain Res Bull,* 16: 33-8, 1986.

126.   SPROUSE JS, AGHAJANIAN GK. (-)-Propranolol blocks the inhibition of serotonergic dorsal raphe cell firing by 5-HT1A selective agonists. *Eur J Pharmacol,* 128: 295-8, 1986.

127.   STARON RS, HIKIDA RS, HAGERMAN FC, DUDLEY GA, MURRAY TF. Human skeletal muscle fiber type adaptability to various workloads. *J Histochem Cytochem,* 32: 146-52, 1984.

128.   STEWART KJ. Exercise training and the cardiovascular consequences of type 2 diabetes and hypertension: plausible mechanisms for improving cardiovascular health. *JAMA,* 288: 1622-31, 2002.

129.   SWAIN RA, HARRIS AB, WIENER SC, DUTKA MV, MORRIS HD, THEIEN BE, KONDA S, ENGBERG K; LAUTERBUR PC, GREENOUGH WT. Prolonged exercise induces angiogenesis and increases cerebral blood volume in primary cortex of the rat. *Neuroscience,* 117:1037-46, 2003.

130.   SZOSTAK C, JAKUBOVIC A, PHILLIPS AG, FIBIGER HC. Bilateral augmentation of dopaminergic and serotonergic activity in the striatum and nucleus accumbens induced by conditioned circling. *J Neurosci,* 6: 2037-44, 1986.

131.   TABER E, BRODAL A, WALBERG F. The raphe nuclei of the brainstem in the cat. I. Normal topography and cytoarchitecture and general discussion. *J Comp Neurol,* 114: 161-87, 1960.

132.   TAKASE LF, BARONE JR, NOGUEIRA MI. Involvement of the caudal raphe nuclei in the feeding behavior of rats. *Braz J Med Biol Res,* 33: 223-8, 2000.

133.   TALMADGE RJ, ROY RR, EDGERTON R. Muscle fiber types and function. *Curr Opin Rheumatol,* 5: 695-705, 1993.

134.   TISCHLER RC, MORIN LP. Reciprocal serotonergic connections between the hamster median and dorsal raphe nuclei. *Brain Res,* 981: 126-32, 2003.

135.   TONG L, SHEN H, PERREAU VM, BALAZS R, COTMAN CW. Effects of exercise on gene-expression profile in the rat hippocampus. *Neurobiol Dis,* 8: 1046-56, 2001.

136.   BAKER KG, HALLIDAY GM, TÖRK I, Cytoarchitecture of the human dorsal raphe nucleus. *J Comp Neurol,* 301: 147-61, 1990.

137.   TORK I. Raphe nuclei and serotonin containing systems. In G. Paxinos (ed.). The rat Nervous system. Sidney: Academic Press, pp. 43-78, 1985.

138.   U.S. Department of Health and Human Services, Physical activity and Health: a report of the Surgeon General. Atlanta: National Center for Chronic Disease Prevention and Health Promotion, 1996.

139. VERTES RP, KOCSIS B. Projections of the dorsal raphe nucleus to the brainstem: PHA-L analysis in the rat. *J Comp Neurol*, 340: 11-26, 1994.

140. VOGLER C, BOVE KE. Morphology of skeletal muscle in children. An assessment of normal growth and differentiation. *Arch Pathol Lab Med*, 109: 238-42, 1985.

141. VRBOVÁ G. Influence of activity on some characteristics properties of slow and fast mammalian muscles. *Exerc Sport Sci Rev*, 7: 181-213, 1979.

142. WANG QP, NAKAI Y. The dorsal raphe: an important nucleus in pain modulation. *Brain Res Bull*, 34: 575-85, 1994.

143. WATT B, GROVE R. Perceived exertion: antecedents and applications. *Sports Med*, 15: 225-41, 1993.

144. WATT EW, BUSKIRK ER, PLOTNICKI BA. A comparison of single vs. multiple daily training regimens: some physiological considerations. *Res Q*, 44: 119-23, 1973.

145. WELLS CL. Physical activity and women's health. *Physical Activity and Fitness Research Digest*, 2: 1-6, 1996.

146. WILLIAMS PL, WARWICK R, DYSON M, BANNISTER LH. Gray's Anatomy. 37th ed. London: Churchill Livingstone, 1989.

147. XIE YF, LIU CY, LIU JZ. Nucleus raphe obscurus participates in regulation of gallbladder motility through vagus and sympathetic nerves in rabbits. *Chin J Physiol*, 45: 101-7, 2002.

148. YARASHESKI KE, TEBAS P, STANERSON B, CLAXTON S, MARIN D, BAE K, KENNEDY M, TANTISIRIWAT W, POWDERLY WG. Resistance exercise training reduces hypertriglyceridemia in HIV-

infected men treated with antiviral therapy. *J Appl Physiol*, 90: 133-8, 2001.

Abbreviature list

RLi, rostral linear nucleus of the raphe

CLi, caudal linear nucleus of the raphe

DR, Dorsal raphe nucleus

MnR, median raphe nucleus

PMnR, paramedian raphe nucleus

PnR, pontine raphe nucleus

RMg, magnus raphe nucleus

RPa, pallidus raphe nucleus

ROb, raphe obscurus nucleus

DRC, dorsal raphe nucleus, caudal part

DRD, dorsal raphe nucleus, dorsal part

DRVL, dorsal raphe nucleus, ventrolateral part

DRV, dorsal raphe nucleus, ventral part

DRI, dorsal raphe nucleu, interfascicular subnucleus part

Aq, aqueduct (Sylvius)

mlf, medial longitudinal fasciculus

xscp, decussation of the superior cerebellar peduncle

GiA, gigantocellular reticular nucelus, alpha part

ts, tectospinal tract

py, pyramidal tract

IR, immunoreactive

Trp, tryptophan

f-Trp, free tryptophan

BCAAs, branched-chain amino acids

5-HT, serotonin

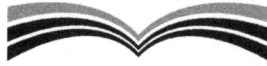

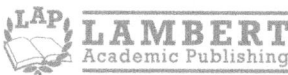

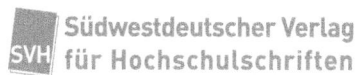

Made in the USA
Las Vegas, NV
30 November 2021